NATIONAL INSTITUTE SOCIAL
SERVICES LIBRARY

Volume 31

THE ADOPTED CHILD
COMES OF AGE

T0262823

THE ADOPTED CHILD
COMES OF AGE

LOIS RAYNOR

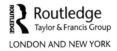
Routledge
Taylor & Francis Group

LONDON AND NEW YORK

First published in 1980 by George Allen & Unwin Ltd

This edition first published in 2022
by Routledge
4 Park Square, Milton Park, Abingdon, Oxon OX14 4RN
605 Third Avenue, New York, NY 10017

Routledge is an imprint of the Taylor & Francis Group, an informa business

British Library Cataloguing in Publication Data
A catalogue record for this book is available from the British Library

ISBN: 978-1-03-203381-5 (Set)
ISBN: 978-1-00-321681-0 (Set) (ebk)
ISBN: 978-1-03-206568-7 (Volume 31) (hbk)
ISBN: 978-1-03-206572-4 (Volume 31) (pbk)
ISBN: 978-1-00-320284-4 (Volume 31) (ebk)

DOI: 10.4324/9781003202844

Publisher's Note
The publisher has gone to great lengths to ensure the quality of this reprint but points out that some imperfections in the original copies may be apparent.

Disclaimer
The publisher has made every effort to trace copyright holders and would welcome correspondence from those they have been unable to trace.

The Adopted Child Comes of Age

LOIS RAYNOR

London
GEORGE ALLEN & UNWIN
Boston   Sydney

GEORGE ALLEN & UNWIN LTD
40 Museum Street, London WC1A 1LU

British Library Cataloguing in Publication Data

Raynor, Lois
    The adopted child comes of age. – (National Insitute for Social Work. Social services library).
    1. Adoption – Great Britain – Case studies
    2. Parent and child – Great Britain – Case studies
    301.42'7   HV887.G5   79-41348

ISBN 0-04-362029-9
ISBN 0-04-362030-2 Pbk

Typeset in 10 on 11 point Times by V & M Graphics Ltd, Aylesbury, Bucks and printed in Great Britain
by Unwin Brothers Ltd, Old Woking, Surrey

CONTENTS

◆

FOREWORD

All of us who have been involved in adoption placements – whether as social workers, case committee members, medical advisers or magistrates – must often have greatly desired to know how these man-made families have worked out. The responsibility of adoption work can at times seem overwhelming, the folklore pervasive, the facts all too few. Anxiously we have asked ourselves whether we are providing for these children the security, happiness and opportunities which their mothers sought when they entrusted them to us? Are our agency policies and procedures the best we can devise? Are the matters we consider important really the crucial issues or ought we to be concentrating on others?

In the half-century since legal adoption was made possible in Britain, more than half a million adoption orders have been granted. This very large-scale placement of children appears to be over, although several thousand babies are still placed for adoption each year along with an increasing number of older children. In addition there are the needs of the existing families to be considered. There is therefore no doubt about the relevance of this study to the present scene even though the situation has changed quite dramatically in some respects.

This is the first study anywhere in the world which has managed to include a really substantial number of adopted adults selected in a systematic way and to consider their responses alongside those of their adoptive parents. The adoptees emerge very creditably from this scrutiny. The majority are evidently confident and capable individuals quite successfully making their way in the world. For the most part they combine loyalty to their adoptive parents with understanding of their birth parents and sensitivity to the feelings and dilemmas which both sets of parents had to face. Overall, their attitudes seem remarkably generous, open and mature.

The four members of the project staff encompassed between them a most impressive range of social work experience gained on both sides of the Atlantic. They set out to seek information needed by social work colleagues all over the world who are similarly engaged in what Jean Charnley so aptly described as 'the art of child placement'. Their knowledge of the subject enabled them to ask the right questions and their careful common sense in interpreting the answers results in a convincing portrayal and discussion of the adoptive experience.

'Success' in adoption cannot be properly measured for there is no yardstick. In fostering we have usually considered a placement successful if it lasts. Much, much more than this is expected of adoption. Indeed, anything less than an apparently perfect outcome has sometimes been termed a failure. Since prediction of any human outcome is notoriously difficult and unreliable, it is of course entirely unrealistic to suppose that happy/successful placements can be guaranteed no matter how excellent the work. Nor is it sensible to equate problems with failure. If the children had been able to remain with their original families, their lives would not have been problem-free either. Nevertheless, if adoption is to be seen as an appropriate way of helping a wider range of deprived, unwanted and handicapped children, it must prove itself on the basis of the eventual outcome of these placements.

On the whole the study findings are reassuring. They tend to confirm rather than upset the basis of present-day practices – indeed, they reaffirm the importance of some long-established ideas which have recently been questioned or even tossed aside as irrelevant. There are frustrations because lack of data in the records made it impossible for the study team to follow up some of their questions. No doubt some people will be disappointed because the clear-cut answers which would simplify decision-making cannot be forthcoming in a subject as complex and individualistic as adoptive family life. But the work done by Miss Raynor and her colleagues and reported here with a wealth of illustration adds to our knowledge, dispels some myths, confirms some hunches and generally sheds light in dark corners. It reaffirms the marvellous capacity of children to overcome a difficult start in life and of loving and sensible adults to become effective parents to a child not born to them. At the same time, this study makes it all too clear that adoption is neither a simple nor an 'ideal' solution.

Among the 164 placements described here there are some sad stories, distressed individuals and failed expectations. Nevertheless it is most encouraging to learn that such a large proportion of those who had been adopted felt it had been a satisfactory experience, that even judged by some fairly stringent criteria, most of them could be considered well-adjusted young adults and that so many of those who had chosen to become adoptive parents were glad they had done so and would recommend this form of parenthood to others.

JANE ROWE

ACKNOWLEDGEMENTS

This study owes much to various people who have contributed their respective knowledge or skills. Most of all, it is indebted to the adopted people who patiently tried to tell us what it had been like to grow up as an adopted child, and to the parents who relived for us the satisfactions and disappointments of their own personal experience in parenting these children. My warmest thanks to all of them for so generously sharing those memories for the benefit of future adoptive families.

Tribute should be paid to the governors of the Thomas Coram Foundation for Children for sponsoring the research; also to the Foundation's director and secretary, J. G. B. Swinley and his staff, for tolerating a major research project in the midst of their regular services to children, and to Miss E. M. Marshall, former children's officer at the Foundation, for her support and encouragement at every stage. To Lady Glover, chairman of the National Adoption Society, and her committee and staff, most sincere thanks are due for their willingness to co-operate in the research.

Sound advice was gratefully received from Dr Michael Humphrey of St George's Hospital Medical School and from Sandra Mason, freelance consultant and former senior research officer at the London Graduate School of Business, who acted as research consultants. Sarah Curtis, editor of *Adoption and Fostering*, Diana Rawstron, secretary to the Legal Group of the Association of British Adoption and Fostering Agencies, and Sally Hamwee, legal advisor to Parents for Children, all read and commented helpfully on the manuscript.

Penelope Layton, Joyce Rae and Robert Tod, the research interviewers, brought to the project not only a wealth of experience in child care but also a keen awareness of the urgent need to add to the body of knowledge about the long-term outcome in adoptions. I am most grateful for their commitment to the study and for their many constructive suggestions. Three other members of the Thomas Coram Foundation staff deserve special thanks for their stalwart service to the study: Phyllis Manning, whose imagination and persistence enabled us to locate so many of the adoptive families after a gap of some twenty years, Jessica Pope, for clerical help in compiling the data and Violet Hopwood, for expert typing of the manuscript.

L.R.

PART ONE

---◆---

LOOKING BACK ON ADOPTION

Chapter 1

---◆---

ADOPTION IN RETROSPECT

This book is about the adoptive experience as it appears in retrospect to young adults who were adopted as children and as it is perceived by their adoptive parents. The information is based on a project undertaken and carried out by the Thomas Coram Foundation for Children and largely funded by that organisation. The aims of the project were to compare the experience of families where children had been adopted by foster parents with others where the children had been received directly for adoption, and to learn something about the role played by various other factors in the long-term outcome of the placements.

Questions galore arise even among professionals when adoption is discussed. What is the nature of adoptive family life over the years and what does it mean to those personally involved in it? What are its satisfactions and disappointments? How do adopted people feel about the family they were given, the opportunities they were offered? Do they fulfil their adoptive parents' expectations? Are they reasonably happy and well-adjusted adults? Does it really matter whether the adoption grew out of a fostering relationship or was a permanent arrangement right from the start? For years, placement agencies have counselled parents to tell the child of his adoptive status, but even now too little is known of how or when adopted children actually learn that they once had other parents. In fact, much of adoption theory and practice is still based on impressions gathered from the limited experience of individual social workers or on follow-up studies made early in the family's life together. Later, the people who could answer these questions, that is, the grown-up adopted people themselves and their adoptive parents, have seldom been asked because of the difficulty of finding a sample that could be studied systematically.

The Thomas Coram Foundation for Children was particularly interested in learning how foster parent adoptions turn out, since its work had resulted in a good many such adoptions. It seemed that these families might be willing to share their experiences for the benefit of future adoptive families, thus making a systematic study possible. The Foundation, formerly known as the Foundling Hospital, had been a real pioneer in fostering, as it had boarded out babies from the Hospital from its inception over 200 years ago. Indeed, the famous eighteenth-century artist and benefactor of the Hospital

William Hogarth and his wife were fostering some of the foundlings at the time of Hogarth's death in 1764. Until modern times the children were boarded out only until they were 5 years old; then they were returned to the Hospital for education and training. When the Hospital finally discontinued institutional care, children were boarded out indefinitely unless their original mothers made a successful application to reclaim them, but beginning in 1947 some of the children began to be legally adopted by their foster parents.

In 1972, when the Foundation registered as an adoption society, over 500 foster children had already been legally adopted with the tacit approval of the agency and the active work of foster parents in securing the consent of the natural mothers. When it was found that more than 130 of those who had been legally adopted were now over 21 years old, the Foundation felt these young adults and the people who had adopted them, if they could be found after so many years, might be willing to take part in a study of how these adoptions had turned out. By sharing the recollection of their own personal experiences they could benefit many children in the future whose long-term care would be planned jointly by social agencies and natural parents. Many children in Britain and elsewhere continue to be placed with people who initially only plan to foster them, but later adopt them if natural parents give their consent. The number of such adoptions may increase, since the Children Act, 1975, now makes it possible for people who have fostered a child for five years to apply to the court for an adoption order without the placing agency necessarily agreeing to the plan. Little is known about how foster parent adoptions turn out, whether they are more, or less, satisfactory for adoptive parents and children in the long term than direct adoption in which natural parents are prepared to relinquish their rights and responsibilities and the adopters are prepared to commit themselves fully as parents to the child right from the start.

The Thomas Coram project with the author as its director was carried out by social workers primarily for other social workers and the families and children they serve. These are some of the questions the project originally sought to answer.

Is adopting one's foster child more or less satisfying and rewarding than adopting a child directly from an adoption agency?

Does being placed first as a foster child affect the long-term satisfaction or adult adjustment of the adoptee?

When there are long delays in legalising the adoption, does this affect the satisfaction of adopters or the satisfaction and adult adjustment of the adoptee?

What is the effect on the adoptive family of contact between birth parents and adoptive parents, for example, during a period of fostering prior to adoption?

If the adoptive experience is satisfying to the parents is it likely to be satisfying to the adoptee as well?

Are adopters and adoptees who perceive themselves as alike in some respects more often satisfied with their experience than those who see no such similarities?

Are the method and timing of the revelation of the child's adoptive status important factors in his adult adjustment?

Are adopted people wanting to meet their birth parents usually those who are not satisfied with their experience in the adoptive family or not well adjusted as adults?

Are parents likely to blame heredity when an adopted child shows behaviour or personality problems while growing up?

Have things which social workers have traditionally considered important proved to be so?

As plans for a study progressed, the possibility of exploring additional aspects of adoptive family life led the project down various paths, some more rewarding than others, but all mainly concerned with family relationships, expectations and achievements.

Chapter 2

---◆---

EARLIER FOLLOW-UP RESEARCH IN ADOPTION

Child adoption is a subject which captures the imagination and a good deal has been written about it in recent years. Much of this has been based on a personal experience of adopting or being adopted, but some of it has been written after long experience of placing children for adoption or as the result of research. The research has tended to be concerned with the relative importance of heredity and environment, the development and adjustment of adopted children and the isolation of factors important in predicting success or failure in adoption. With a few exceptions the research has taken place while the children were still young, usually before adolescence. Research involving *adult* adoptees is still quite limited.

The earliest studies were concerned with how well adopted children had been able to overcome early deprivation and the poor backgrounds from which they had been 'rescued'. Would environment triumph over heredity and a poor start in life? The earliest follow-up research into the long-term outcome of adoption was Sophie Theis's well-known American study *How Foster Children Turn Out*, published in 1924. This study involved all the children who had been placed by the New York State Charities Aid Association (a voluntary agency), who were between 18 and 40 years old when the study was made and who could be located – nearly 800 in all. Many had come from very 'undesirable' backgrounds or had led very deprived lives before being placed, often as school-aged children. They and their foster parents were interviewed and agency case records consulted.

Theis concluded that many children from 'very undesirable backgrounds (drunkenness, criminality, mental illness, etc.)' were able to take advantage of opportunities when these were offered, and classifying her subjects on the basis of how well they were managing their lives as adults she found nearly three-quarters of them 'capable', which she defined as 'law-abiding, managing their affairs with good sense and living in accordance with good moral standards in their communities'. The 'incapable' were those who were 'unable or unwilling to support themselves adequately, who were shiftless or had defied the accepted standards of morality or order in their communities'. Adoption was very new in New York then and less than one-third of these foster children had been legally adopted, but it was found that this one-third tended to be better educated than the others and more often they had taken some kind of vocational training and therefore had some definite means of self-support. The fact of the legal adoption and that more of them had been placed with these parents before the age of 5 years were both thought to have contributed to this good result.

Further detailed research into the outcome of adoptions came 25 years later with the work of Skodak, Skeels and Harms, published in 1948 and 1949. This, too, was an American study and was concerned with mental development and its relation to the intelligence and educational achievement of parents. Adoption offered a situation in which this could be studied. 'Orphanage infants, who had uneducated parents and poor backgrounds' and had been placed for adoption before they were 6 months old, were followed up with repeated interviews with adoptive parents and intelligence tests on the children until the children averaged 13 years of age. The intellectual development and educational achievement of their adoptive parents were studied too. At 5 years of age the children's intellectual development equalled or exceeded the mean of the general population. Although as the children grew older a limit to mental development seemed to be set by heredity, their mean IQ at age 13 was still some 20 points higher than their birth mother's IQ. From these findings it appeared that the development of intelligence could be modified very considerably by environment but within limits which had been established for the individual by his inheritance. The personal qualities of the adoptive parents were found to be very important to the mental growth of children as well as to their emotional stability.

During the decade of the 1950s adoption became much more widespread in both Britain and the United States, and those responsible for placing the children were keen to learn what factors or conditions were required for a successful outcome and whether such an outcome could be predicted. Two studies were published in Britain, one in 1953 by Lulie Shaw, who had interviewed 55 sets of Quaker parents when their adopted children were under 10 years old, and one by Robina Addis et al. in 1955, based on adoption agency records. During the same decade Ruth Brenner (1951) was following up children placed by the Free Synagogue Child Adoption Committee in New York City, and in 1957 Dr J. R. Wittenborn was following up another group at Yale University's Child Development Clinic. Both Brenner and Wittenborn were particularly interested in psychological tests in predicting later development. Working with a team of child psychologists, psychiatrists and social workers Wittenborn studied a group of adopted children aged 5 and 6 and another group aged 8 to 9 years, who had been given Gesell developmental tests in infancy and were tested again during the study. The later IQ was found to be related to the education and ambitions of the adoptive parents and to some extent to the occupational level of the birth parents, but Wittenborn concluded that 'much of the effort commonly devoted to an exact evaluation of infants considered for adoption could more profitably be devoted to a study of the applicants who desire to be adoptive parents'. Brenner, too, was disillusioned with the predictive value of infant tests and found the qualities of the adoptive parents much more important.

The 1960s saw several more follow-up undertakings, as well as some clinical studies and considerable interest in adoption theory and practice. In Florida Helen Witmer and her colleagues (1963) carried out a study which described how families who had adopted children privately in the State of Florida appeared to be functioning ten years later. Witmer found the families functioning satisfactorily in 70 per cent of the cases, with girls making a better adjustment than boys. Compared with a group of natural children the adopted children, both boys and girls, appeared to be at a slight disadvantage in personal and social functioning but not in intelligence or school achievement.

A little later, Bryn Mawr College and the Children's Aid Society of Pennsylvania conducted a joint research project involving a random sample of 250 white children, median age 9½ years, who had been adopted through the Children's Aid Society (Lawder *et al.*, Vol. I, 1969, and Hoopes *et al.*, Vol. II, 1970). The children's behaviour was rated by means of interviews with adoptive parents and also by use of an adjustment rating scale devised for teachers and through personality measurement tests on the children. About 73 per cent of the families were rated as good or superior, and the children showed no more pathology than the natural-born children in a matched control group. The achievement of the majority of the adopted children was rated as 'good' but not so many children were rated 'excellent' as in the control group. No significant differences, such as might have been expected on the basis of practice theory, were found between the adopted children and the natural children.

At the same time that these studies were being made in the United States, Alexina McWhinnie (1967) and Margaret Kornitzer (1968) published follow-up studies in Britain. Dr McWhinnie's Scottish research was the first since the Theis study more than 40 years before to use adopted people's own experience of adoption in a systematic way. This study sought to learn how adoption was experienced by the persons ultimately most concerned, what problems they met, whether there were recurring patterns in the adoption situation, and whether there were particular environmental factors which had been conducive to good adjustment and others to poor adjustment. Guided interviews were conducted with 58 adults (14 men and 44 women) aged 18 to 60, who had been placed as children, and all but 6 of them adopted. This 'unselected sample' was procured from family doctors who referred to the project any patient they knew was adopted and who was willing to be interviewed in the project. McWhinnie classified the adjustment of the 52 adoptees as 'Good' (15), 'Fairly Good' (6), 'Intermediate' (21), 'Poor' (10). This was the first time information had been gleaned from adopted people themselves about how their adoptive status had been revealed to them, whether they were curious to know more about their biological parents and how free they had felt to discuss the subject with the adopters. McWhinnie concluded that a child should be told by his adoptive parents before the age of 5 and that the whole area of communication between adoptive parents and children was fraught with emotional implications.

Margaret Kornitzer (1968) interviewed 664 adoptive families secured from five different English sources. Many were *de facto* adoptions, i.e. never legalised, and the adopted people ranged in age from under 5 years to 70. She had found it impossible to obtain a good cross-section of adopted adults, so although some 62 adults were included, most of her data relate to an undifferentiated age group, where she assessed about three-quarters as 'successful' or 'reasonably successful' adoptions. She found many adopters 'heavily infected by their fears of heredity and subconsciously waiting for trouble'. She saw adoption surrounded by self-deception and even mental and emotional dishonesty, and she thought problems and difficulties were often related to this. She believed that relationships within the adoptive family would be better if there were less secrecy and evasion, and that the time had come to consider how adopted people could be given the right to learn essential knowledge about their origins.

Research into adoption outcome became more popular in the 1970s and included follow-up studies of transracial adoption in Britain (Raynor, 1970; Jackson, 1975) and in the United States (Fanshel, 1972; Grow and Shapiro, 1974; Simon and Altstein, 1977) and a study of children placed when older (Kadushin, 1970). These findings were encouraging, as cases in which children had been placed transracially or when older showed a satisfactory outcome in just about the same proportions as had been found in the follow-up studies of white baby placements, and the problems around racial identity for children placed across racial lines had not materialised.

There also were studies of more conventional placements in Sweden, Britain and the United States during this decade. The Swedish research (Bohman, 1970) explored a representative group of adopted children and their families about 10 years after their placement by the welfare committee of Stockholm City. It was hoped to learn something about the factors relative to harmonious development of adoptive families. It was found that 'neither the factors that were known about the biological parents, the pre- or perinatal circumstances, the child's age at placement nor the factors studied concerning the adoptive home provided a sufficient explanation for the variations in the children's behaviour'.

A somewhat similar study was carried out in England by the National Children's Bureau as part of its National Child Development Study (Seglow *et al.*, 1972). As part of the larger study, these adopted children could be compared with the whole cohort of children of the same age in the general population and also with illegitimate children kept by their mothers. By the age of 7, when this study was made, the adopted children had overcome their earlier handicap of illegitimacy and were achieving more in school and making a better adjustment there than the illegitimate children of the same age who had been kept by their mothers, and they also compared favourably with their peers in the general population. The findings indicated the important influence of the environment on the children's development and led to the conclusion that we can have considerable confidence in adoption. A study of these same children at the age of 11 has now been undertaken by the National Children's Bureau.

Another Engish study (Tizard, 1977) assessed children who had spent the first two to seven years of their lives in an institution, and compared the 30 who were later adopted with the 23 who were restored to their birth parents or fostered on a long-term basis. At age 8 most of the adoptions were considered 'successful', judged by a number of different criteria. When they were compared with the alternative placements available to them, that is, continued institutional care, long-term fostering, or restoration to the natural families they had never really known, Tizard found adoption 'clearly the best solution to the child's needs'.

Two early studies of grown-up adoptees, one by Theis and the other by McWhinnie, have already been mentioned. Two further major studies of adult adopted people were published in the 1970s – one in America (Jaffee and Fanshel, 1970) and one in Britain (Triseliotis, 1973).

Jaffee and Fanshel studied the life adjustment of 100 adult adoptees, aged 20 to 30, who had been placed by one of four participating agencies in New York City and who were found still living in the area. All the children were Caucasian and under 3 years of age when placed in their adoptive homes. This retrospective research aimed to provide for adoption agencies a picture of families who had brought up their children with relative success and satisfaction, as well as those where the child's life had been unhappy or problematic. Many aspects of family life over the years were examined. An attempt was made to measure the outcome of the adoptive experience and to assess the adoptees' life situation at the time of follow-up. Some adoptees had encountered quite serious adjustment problems, but many others had shown 'remarkably few' problems, past or present. No attempt was made to shed light upon the differences that might exist between adoptive families and other families.

How they Fared in Adoption (Jaffee and Fanshel, 1970) reports the findings from Fanshel's interviews with the adoptive parents. Unfortunately, only about half the families agreed to their adoptee taking part in the research, and in the event only one-third were interviewed. The complete findings from even those 33 interviews have not been published, although they have been recorded in a doctoral dissertation and certain aspects of the study appeared in *Child Welfare* (1974, vol. 53, no. 4).

Because of the Scottish legal provision for adoptee access to birth records after the age of 17, Scotland was the setting for Dr Triseliotis' study (1973) of 70 adult adoptees who had been in touch with Register House in Edinburgh for information from their original birth registrations. The adoptees were interviewed with the aim of identifying the general circumstances of adopted adults who had sought information about their origins, and to establish their reasons for the search, and how they had used the information after they got it. Interviews revealed that the impulse to search was in response to some deeply felt psychological need.

Triseliotis identified two groups with different search goals – those who wanted to find one or both natural parents and those who wished only to obtain information. Those who hoped to find their natural parents were much more strongly motivated and more determined than those who were only seeking information. Where the adoptees perceived their life with the adopters as unsatisfactory they often had a poor self-concept, and the greater the dissatisfaction with their family relationships and with themselves, the more likely they were to be searching for their birth parents and not just seeking information about them. Triseliotis concluded from his research that the quest for origins was an attempt by adopted persons to understand themselves and their situation better and that no person should be cut off from his origins.

From these studies we see how attitudes to adoption have changed over the last 50 years in Britain and the United States. From a rescue operation for children of all ages with poor backgrounds and early experience of neglect or abuse, adoption soon became a resource largely for 'blue ribbon' babies who could satisfy the longings and requirements of infertile couples. Interest in research shifted to the relative influence of heredity and environment, especially upon mental development, and the possibility of predicting the 'success' or 'failure' of these infant placements. The strong influence of environment, most of all the attitudes of the adoptive parents, led social workers and the public to greater confidence in adoption not only for healthy white infants but even for older children and for children placed transracially. Most recently, feedback from adopted people themselves via research caused growing concern about adoptees being denied the right to know something of their origins, and this concern led to the provision in the 1975 Children Act for adopted persons over the age of 18 to have access to their original birth certificate after counselling.

Researchers have found that adoption is complex, that there are few easy answers to the many questions it precipitates. So many factors are involved in adoption, in so many possible combinations, that it is not surprising to find the results of research not all in agreement and often without any very firm conclusions. The Thomas Coram Foundation study is being reported here as a contribution to the body of knowledge gradually being built up on adoption.

Chapter 3

DESIGN OF THIS STUDY

This project was planned as a descriptive and analytical inquiry based on separate interviews with adult adopted persons and their adoptive parents, and systematic examination of the information contained in the case records of these people. It was decided that the families to be studied should consist of the entire group of 133 families who fostered a child for the Thomas Coram Foundation (TCF) – a Caucasian child born in England or Wales between 1948 and 1951 inclusive – and later adopted this child who would be 22 to 27 years old at the time of the interviews. Starting with those born in 1948, the first year in which any appreciable number of the foster children was legally adopted, we worked forward to those born in 1951 who were 21 in 1972 when the project was being set up.

Through the co-operation of the National Adoption Society (NAS) a comparison group was made available for study. These were families who had adopted directly through that agency in the usual way and had taken a Caucasian child born in England or Wales between 1948 and 1951. At the time the children were placed with them these families all lived in the same sections of England as the foster parent adopters, that is, London, the Home Counties and East Anglia. It was thought that cultural differences in other parts of the country might possibly affect adoption outcome, so this additional factor was avoided. As there were over 200 such placements by the National Adoption Society, the cases were arranged in date order and every third case was eliminated, leaving 155 families for the study. With the 133 from the Thomas Coram Foundation this gave a total of 288 families (and children) to be included if they could be found and if they were willing to take part in the research.

Where two adopted children in a family fell within the age group, these cases were listed in order by case number and in the first such case the elder of the two children in the age group was selected for the study, in the second case the younger was selected, and so on down the list of families who had two adopted children born in the years covered by the survey. As planned, the two agencies were considered separately when comparing the two methods by which children had been received into their families. Later they were combined for the advantages of larger numbers for a study of various factors in relation to adoption outcome as such, where the method of placement seemed of minor importance. It is this combined group which is the subject of this book except as otherwise noted.

Comprehensive code books were set up to receive the information from the case records and from the interviews in a form suitable for use on a computer. Next, the case records pertaining to the 288 families and children selected for study were read and the information was coded. This was followed by the arduous task of locating the families, then reopening agency contact with them after a gap of up to 25 years. The original selection was reduced, first by those who had died, emigrated, or simply could not be found, and later by those who were located but were unwilling to participate. The interviews took place with the remainder, first with the adoptive parents and then by separate appointment with the adult adoptees. After each interview the material was entered in the appropriate code book. When all the interviews had been completed, it was the computer's task to provide the figures for analysis and interpretation.

USING THE CASE RECORDS

One of the limitations of research involving old case records is that they are likely to be short on facts and even more sketchy on feelings, and these records were no exception. This placed serious limitations on any effort to explore possible links between later adjustment and a child's genetic background or his early experience of life before this placement. It restricted our knowledge of the emotional climate in the family when the child entered it, as there was very seldom any mention of such important information as the personality of the adoptive parents, the warmth of family relationships, the attitude to their childlessness or inability to have further natural children, their feelings about illegitimacy and a child's birth parents. An important and emotive subject such as the adopters' attitude to their infertility, which apparently had not been discussed at the time of the adoption application, was not included in the project, as it could hardly be raised now for the first time, in a single research interview. No criticism of the earlier work is intended, since quite naturally practice has changed over 20 to 30 years and will continue to do so.

In spite of the scarcity of recorded attitudes and feelings, most case records contained some factual information about the children, their birth mothers and the adoptive parents. Very little was recorded about putative fathers. Facts about the children included their sex – 176 boys and 112 girls [61 per cent boys, 39 per cent girls] their birth weight, the length of time they had been with their birth mothers and how many placements they had had in foster homes and residential nurseries; their age when placed with these adopters and their age when the adoptive orders were made. Useful facts about the biological parents included in most cases only the age and occupation of the mothers and sometimes the occupation of the maternal grandfathers. Concerning the adoptive parents their age and occupation were recorded, along with the age of other children already in the family; the type of community, accommodation and housekeeping standards; how the children settled, their early feelings about them, and whether they had met the natural mothers. These facts were recorded consistently enough to be useful, but such details about the child and his biological parents as length of gestation, illnesses during pregnancy, perinatal condition, education and health history of the mothers and fathers were all recorded too infrequently to be of much use in the study. In the cases of direct adoption an agency worker did not visit after the placement, this being left to the welfare supervisor and the guardian *ad litem*. This meant that the only information about the children's health, development and behaviour during the period they were in the family before legal adoption was whatever the adopters saw fit to mention to the agency in their letters. As they were anxious that all should be seen to be going along well so there would be no delay in the granting of an adoption order, there were almost no reports of any difficulties with these young children during the first months when they were settling into their new homes.

FINDING THE FAMILIES

The search for a total of 288 families, most of whom had not been heard from in up to 25 years, proved a formidable task, especially as it was necessary to do it confidentially. Eventually, just over three-quarters of them were found to be living in England where they could be interviewed if they were willing. Another ten had emigrated or were living abroad temporarily and in five other cases both parents were known to have died.

Extensive use was made of telephone directories and the task would have been simplified if everyone were on the telephone. Electoral rolls served to verify an address found in some other way or for following up a lead; in fact, an address was not considered found until verified in the current electoral roll, as it was important that a letter about the project should not fall into the hands of anyone except the adoptive parents.

The first step was to check the family's last known address with their local telephone directory and the electoral rolls. If they were not on the telephone at this address the same and other directories were searched. This called for some knowledge of population movements as well as much scanning of telephone directories. Others were located through such sources as professional directories, *Kelly's Directory*, death registrations, the marriage registrations of adoptees, solicitors who handled the adoption, referees and relatives known to the agency at the time of placement, or a combination of more than one of these. Some were found despite their having moved more than once since the last agency contact with them. Hardest to find were people whose last known address was in an area which had been redeveloped. No one, even their local council, seemed to know where these people had gone and they were the very ones least likely to be on the telephone. It may be that some of these parents, too, had died or emigrated (Table 3.1).

Table 3.1 *Result of search for adoptive families*

	Located in England	Abroad	Died	Not Found	Total
TCF	103	6	3*	21	133
NAS	120	4	2	29	155
Total	223	10	5	50	288

*There was a fourth case where both parents had died but an adoptive relative who brought up the child was interviewed.

PARENTS WHO REFUSED

Of the 223 families who were located, 63 refused the invitation to take part in the research, leaving 160 to be interviewed. This was an acceptance rate of 72 per cent of those located and available. The response was somewhat better from former foster parents, perhaps because it was their agency which was making the study, with the result that the fostering agency's cases made up 52 per cent of the final group whereas they had comprised only 46 per cent of the original selection.

Table 3.2 *Result of efforts to interview adoptive families*

Not found, died or emigrated	65
Refused to take part	63
Interviewed	160
Original selection	288

When those who were not found or were known to have died or emigrated were added to those who refused to participate, the final number left to be interviewed was 56 per cent of the original number (Table 3.2).

In order to learn how representative these final 160 were of the original 288, they were compared on 10 items on which information was available in the case records. It was reasonable to think that any of these might have been related to willingness to participate in the study or possibly to our ability to locate them. Seven of the items were factual, including sex of the child, age of the child when placed in this family, the child's medical history at placement, age of the adoptive parents, occupation and resulting social class of the adoptive parents, contacts between the adopters and the child's natural family and length of time between placement and legal adoption. The other three were feelings expressed by the adoptive parents about the child before legalisation of the adoption, including any mention of a child's intellectual development or behaviour problems, and whether the child met their wishes as to age, sex, health and appearance when placed with them.

The results of this comparison showed that the families who were interviewed were remarkably like the original overall group on all these items. When the characteristics of the two groups were analysed the respective proportions did not differ by more than 6 per cent and in most cases the differences were much smaller. So on the basis of this early information about the families there is reason to think that the adoptive parents who were interviewed were reasonably representative of the original selection. Because of lack of later information about the families who refused or were not found, they could not be compared systematically with the families who were seen on the basis of more recent events in their lives. However, there were some tantalising bits of information in the letters of refusal and these can be mentioned.

Of the 63 families who refused, one-third simply did not reply to two letters inviting them to take part. Some others wrote briefly to say they preferred not to participate, but some people wrote long letters about their children, while others simply referred to their happiness or disappointment in them. One family wrote that they had never told their child she was adopted, yet some others who had not told did nevertheless take part in the study. This may well have been the real reason for some of the other refusals. Another family were so angry with their agency for the 10 years of uncertainty they had endured until they could adopt the foster child they had taken (at least in their own minds) with a view to adoption that they could not bring themselves to dredge it up again. They were bitter because they believed they had been caught up in an agency disagreement over policy as to whether adoption or return to an unmarried mother should be encouraged for children in foster care. A father said: 'Ours has not been a happy experience and we do not wish to raise spectres of the past.' Another said: 'Some things have happened we would rather forget.'

Whilst some adoptive parents indicated they simply did not wish to be bothered, there were others whose decision not to take part was very understandable. In one case the child had died just a year before and in another the adoptive father had just died. In two other families both parents were very worried about their own extremely poor health. In six cases the adopters' marriage had broken down or they were in such serious conflict that they felt they could not discuss their situation. One father who refused to take part wrote rather callously that he and his former wife had been divorced many years ago and he had no idea where his wife and the child were now.

Although these instances might lead one to think otherwise, actually just as many parents wrote enthusiastically about their child but still were unwilling to take part in the study. It is sometimes assumed that follow-up studies are heavily weighted with successful placements, that those with an unfortunate outcome would refuse to take part in an inquiry. As we have seen, some of these did refuse in this study, but the others took part and even said they had found it helpful to talk about their problems. No doubt there are many individual reasons why some families participate in such studies and others do not, but quite a few of the adoptive families we interviewed told us it had been rather a shock to hear from the agency when the adoption had not been mentioned for years and they had long ago 'forgotten' about it. Could it be that maintaining the fantasy they had built up over the years was the most important thing to some of those who opted out?

THE INTERVIEWS WITH ADOPTIVE PARENTS

The families were all approached by a carefully drafted informal letter signed by the senior officer of their agency, explaining the study was undertaken so that social workers could learn the long-term results of their work of placing children in families and thereby improve the service to future families and children. Parents were invited to take part in the study by being interviewed at a time and place convenient to them. The letters were not all sent at the same time but gradually over the years 1973 to 1975, because it seemed unfair to open up the subject of adoption and then allow time for anxiety to be generated before the letter could be followed up with an interview.

Most of the parents were seen at home and in most cases they welcomed the research worker warmly. Many were interviewed in the evening or at the weekend, but some who were retired could be seen during normal working hours. It was necessary in an interview usually of about two hours' duration to obtain a great deal of information about a very personal subject – facts, feelings and opinions – and to do this without detriment to the people concerned. It was felt that an understanding of adoption, and sensitivity to how far to probe for deeper feelings, were required of interviewers in a study of this kind and called for social work skills of a high order. Three qualified social workers with considerable experience of child care and adoption placement work, and able to make the adjustment to research interviewing, were employed specially for the project on a part-time basis. They had to interpret the study and help families and adoptees to relate to them as gatherers of information rather than as casework helpers. When parents or adoptees wanted information from their case records they were advised to discuss this request with a member of the regular staff at their agency.

One hundred and sixty sets of parents were seen. Of these, 83 were Thomas Coram Foundation cases which had begun as fostering, and 77 were direct adoptions through the National Adoption Society. In 116 of the 160 families both parents were interviewed together. In another 23 only the mother was seen and in 13 others only the father (because only one parent was living or available or in a few cases because only one was willing); in 7 a step-adoptive parent was seen along with the remaining original adoptive parent and in 1 case where both parents had died we saw the adoptive aunt who had brought up the boy. Only two couples chose to be interviewed at the agency office and three fathers at their place of business. In one instance the father, a publican who was divorced and remarried, chose to be interviewed at the bar before opening hours supported by a loud radio and a bottle of sherry. Interviews varied in length from one to four hours and all took place between April 1973 and February 1976.

Content of the adoptive parent interviews
In addition to some demographic information, the interviews focused on the adoptive parents' view of how the adoption had turned out. This included their overall assessment of the experience with this child, their satisfactions and disappointments, their early response to the child and the child's response to them in terms of how he had settled; the advantages or disadvantages of the child having come to them first as a foster child or directly for adoption as the case might be; their attitude to the natural mother; their relationship with the child over the years and how communication with the child about his adoptive status was handled; their description of the child's health and development, behaviour and achievement. Interviewers had a more detailed list of these subjects (see Appendix B) in order to avoid bias in the interviewing and to make the coverage as complete as possible, but they were not required to cover the subjects in any particular order.

The interviews were not structured question-and-answer sessions and there was no note-taking, as almost everyone readily consented to the interviews being taped. Interviewers explained the sort of information the project was interested in, and parents were left to tell their own story in their own way with only occasional unlocking questions from the interviewer and guidance in keeping to the subject matter. For instance, sometimes parents preferred to discuss another of their children instead of the one in the study and had to be reminded which one was included. Perhaps it is not surprising that parents covered most of the subjects with only a little prompting, since most people enjoy talking about their children, and the kind of information the project wanted was largely what people would be likely to include when telling of their life together as a family.

This was a retrospective study and doubtless some of the content would have been different if the research had been done longitudinally over the years, as people tend to forget, especially unpleasant things; but we were interested in how the parents and adopted people felt about these things now that the experience was in the past. What sort of memories had it left them with? Was there a rosy glow over everything now, or could they be more objective now that the children were grown up? It is impossible to know how much enchantment this distance lent to the events of earlier years, but as for remembering, parents often recalled the smallest details of life with their children and all had a vivid recollection of the first time they saw the child and brought him home, the time when a dream had suddenly become the reality of parenting a child who needed them even more than they needed him.

ADOPTEE INTERVIEWS

The project interviewed 105 of the adoptees (56 from the fostering agency and 49 from the adoption agency) including four whose parents had not been interviewed. In two of these four cases both parents had died, but the adoptee when approached about the project wished to participate. In the other two cases the parents refused for themselves but were willing for their sons to take part.

The possibility of interviewing the adopted adult son or daughter was discussed with the parents only after they had had a chance to see at first hand how their own interviews were conducted and had been assured that the research worker would not divulge to the adoptee anything they had said in their interview or, still more important, any information about the adoptee's background. Many parents needed reassurance about the worker's role as a gatherer not a giver of information, and some who ultimately agreed to the adoptee being seen almost certainly would not have permitted it if this had been requested in the letter before contact with the worker. It was usually suggested that the parents themselves might tell their child about the study and leave it to him to decide about participating. It was surprising how many parents who did not want the adult adoptee to take part felt they should make this negative decision for him without consulting his wishes. No matter how well adjusted the son or daughter was said to be, some parents felt he or she was, nevertheless, vulnerable around the subject of adoption and should be protected from any mention of it. It seemed as though they had been protecting their children all their lives from people who were inquisitive about their origins, and they were not about to abandon this parental function now that the children had grown up. At the same time, and perhaps more fundamentally, they protected themselves from the dreadful possibility, which was very real to them in spite of anything we might say, that any discussion of adoption would open some Pandora's box of long-forgotten interest in the children's background.

Seven of the adoptees were not available for interview as they were living abroad. Another had been killed on a motorbike at the age of 17, and one was permanently in hospital as he was severely subnormal. In three cases the parents were out of touch with their sons and did not know where they were living. Four adoptees obviously could not participate in the study since their parents had never told them they were adopted and hoped they still did not know. There were seven cases in which the adopted persons themselves refused an interview, although only one of these refused outright and she was a girl who was described to us as always responding negatively to anything that was asked of her. Two of the seven did not reply to our letters when parents asked us to contact them directly, two girls seemed very lukewarm about the idea and said their husbands would not approve. Two young men showed interest, but also mixed feelings as they arranged several appointments over the period of a year but never quite made it.

The other 36 who were not interviewed had the decision made for them by their parents. Some of the reasons given by adoptive parents for their unwillingness to have a son or daughter take part in the research revealed their insecurity in the role of parents to these children and the doubts and fears they had been keeping locked up out of sight for so many years. They had told the child he was adopted, as they had been advised to do, but when this conflicted with their quite normal wish to make the child their own, they had soft-pedalled adoption and kept any discussion about it to a minimum. One father said 'A word might spark something', and another thought it 'dangerous' and said his daughter had probably forgotten or it had not occurred to her to tell her husband and he might resent it. A parent said: 'It is better not to disturb the subconscious – leave it sleeping.' Other parents said 'Things are best left as they are', or they feared upsetting something which had 'worked out so marvellously'. Several said they thought the adoptee would not even want to hear adoption mentioned or, in fact, would have forgotten all about it.

In some of the families where the project was denied an interview with the adoptee the subject of the adoption had not been mentioned between parents and children for anywhere from 10 to 20 years, so parents understandably felt it could not be raised now. They felt that as long as their children showed no obvious interest in their adoption or background, no interest existed, but that any mention of it was likely to awaken it and they saw this as leading to unhappiness for all concerned. One mother said she wouldn't want her daughter's 'mind to wander' now that she was married and had her own family. Another said the adoption had only been mentioned once, when her son was 7 years old – why should she remind him of it now at 25? In fact, this woman hoped and indeed believed her son had forgotten what he had been told. A father said his boy had been told at the age of 9 and had said he never wanted it mentioned again, so it never had been. In all these cases adoption was clearly a closed subject.

It was important to know if the 105 participating adoptees were representative of the whole 288 in the original selection, and it seemed of interest also to know how they compared with the 160 who would have been seen were it not for the reasons just mentioned. These two comparisons were undertaken.

As the 288 in the original selection included some families who were not interviewed, this analysis had to be limited to factual information from the old case records. The comparison was made on eight items including sex of the adoptee, his age at placement and the length of time between placement and legal adoption, the age of both adoptive parents, their occupation and social class grouping, and contact between them and the child's natural parents. The differences found were so minor that we feel justified in believing that the 105 who were interviewed were indeed representative of the larger group originally selected for study. The sexes were very slightly more evenly divided in the group we saw, where 56 per cent were male compared with 61 per cent in the original group. Somewhat fewer of those interviewed (50 per cent compared with 57 per cent) had been legally adopted during their first year in these families, and somewhat more of them (29 per cent compared with 22 per cent) were in families where there had been some direct contact between the adopters and the natural mother or some member of her family. These last two points may almost certainly be attributed to the larger proportion of children in the participating group who were from the fostering agency.

The second analysis compared the 105 adoptees who were interviewed with the total 160 who might have been seen. They were compared on 10 points on which it would be reasonable to surmise that differences might exist. These items included: the sex of the adoptee; the length of time between placement and legal adoption; social and occupational group of the adoptive parents; basis on which the adoptee was originally received into the family; the adoptive parents' overall satisfaction in their experience with this child; the frequency with which adoption was discussed with the adoptee over the years; how much control the parents felt they had exercised during the growing-up years; the existence of behaviour or personality problems while growing up; parents' assessment of the adoptee's use of the opportunities offered him.

This comparison, too, was remarkable for the similarity between the adoptees available for interview and the whole 160 whose parents had been seen. When the characteristics of the two groups were analysed, the respective proportions did not differ by more than 1 or 2 per cent except in the case of one, where the difference was 6 per cent. This characteristic was the frequency with which the subject of adoption had been discussed in these families over the years. It is reasonable to expect that families who have discussed adoption freely over the years and have made no secret of it would be more willing to have their children take part in such an inquiry than families who have mentioned the subject only once or twice, or as in four cases here, have *never* disclosed the fact of adoption to the child. The idea of opening up the subject after so many years was simply too threatening to some who had always kept a low profile on adoption.

Content of adoptee interviews

Interviews with the young adult adoptees, who by this time were aged 22 to 27, focused on their experience of growing up in the adoptive family and their current personal and social adjustment, including their overall assessment of their experience; their relationship with the adoptive family; their view of parental expectations; the opportunities they were given and the kind of care they recieved; when their adoptive status was revealed to them and their reaction to the revelation; their ease in discussing this with their adoptive parents and their attitude now to their birth parents; their view of themselves, their overall view of life and their satisfaction with their own lives at the present time. These interviews were handled in the same way as those with the parents, that is, they were largely unstructured and no attempt was made to discuss the various aspects of their experiece in any particular order. To avoid bias and ensure coverage interviewers had a list of the subjects to be covered (see Appendix C) and they brought the interview back to these subjects if it ranged too far afield.

CODING THE INFORMATION

The tapes were played back later by the interviewer concerned and by the author who was also the project director. Each coded the information separately, then discussed any differences and, if necessary, listened again to parts of the tape to arrive at a mutually agreed coding. This meant that the project director heard all the interviews with the exception of a very few which could not be taped, and that the detailed codings all involved two people, one of whom had actually seen and interviewed the particular person and one of whom was familiar with every case and could see each one in relation to all the others. This was done in order to overcome any differences in interpretation arising out of the fact that more than one interviewer was involved in the project. The subjects covered in interviews were broken down in the code books into 108 items from the parental interviews and 47 from the adoptee interviews. The difference in the number of items covered reflected to some extent the uncertainty in the social work world about what sort of information might be available from adult adopted people.

ANALYSING THE RESULTS

Although the families and children who were studied were representative of those served by the two agencies concerned, and we had some reason to think they were also fairly typical of British agency adoptions generally in the late 1940s and early 1950s, we were unable to find enough firm information about British adoption placements generally to be able to say that the families in the study were indeed truly representative of British agency placements at that time. Furthermore, since the cases studied were not selected as a random sample of agency placements, strictly speaking tests of statistical significance could not be applied to the results. But since there was no real reason to suppose the placements were atypical, it seemed worthwhile to assess how far the results would have been significant if the sample could have been considered a random one. So chi-square tests of statistical significance were done on the most important areas of analysis and the consequent indications of significance have been taken into account in the comments on the results which follow throughout the text.

Some repetition in reporting is unavoidable because of the inter-relationships between closely related factors which are being examined in different ways. Some of the subjects which appear in Part Two of this book, where they are considered in relation to overall satisfaction and to adult adjustment, are discussed again in Part Three in relation to other factors. All percentages have been rounded to add to 100. All names used are fictitious, and individual cases have been altered in order to preserve anonymity. Guides to the subjects covered in the interviews will be found in the appendixes, and the forms used for coding the information for analysis are available for perusal at the offices of the Thomas Coram Foundation, 40 Brunswick Square, London WC1.

Chapter 4

---◆---

SOME PRELIMINARY DATA

DESCRIPTIVE DATA ON THE FAMILIES AND CHILDREN

Sex of adoptee

Of the adoptive parents who were involved, 92 (57 per cent) had a son in the study and 68 (43 per cent) a daughter. Thus, the ratio of male to female adoptees remained substantially the same as in the original group, where we have seen that it was 61 per cent to 39 per cent, roughly three boys to two girls.

Status of family

In four out of five of the families the adoptive parents were still together, but seven homes had been broken by divorce and there were thirteen in which the father had died and eleven where the mother had died. There also was one already mentioned where both parents had died many years ago but the aunt who had brought up the boy was seen. In two other cases we were able to interview the adoptees even though both parents had died recently and there were no parent substitutes to be interviewed. (In the original group there were three additional cases in which both parents were known to have died, but in these cases there was no way of learning if the adoptees were aware that they were adopted, so the project staff did not feel free to contact them.)

Financial status

Most adoptees were self-supporting or were married women supported by their husbands. Only two were financially dependent on their adoptive parents and one of these was really earning her way, as she kept house for her elderly, widowed father.

Adoptees' marital status

Eighty-eight of the adoptees had been married and seventy-five were still single. In one case the son had left home early and the father and step-mother did not know if he had married. Six of the married had been divorced and half of these had remarried; another thirteen had separated and more often than not the adoptee had returned home to live while a divorce was in progress. The number of divorces, which is 7 per cent of those ever married, can be compared only very roughly with the 1974 official figure of 9 per cent of married couples in the general population of England and Wales, since the latter figure, unlike our own, is for divorcing couples of all ages. Other investigators have found early marriage to be one indicator of divorce and they also have found that the age at which people marry is linked with social class (Gibson, 1974). Thompson and Peretz (eds) (1977) have said: 'The younger the marriage the greater the probability of its ending in divorce.' Most of the failed marriages among our adoptees were early and they appear to have been very ill-advised, as they often lasted without separation for less than a year and in one case only three months. At least one of the young women would certainly be called a battered wife, and another had married a man who very soon afterwards was convicted of assaulting young girls and was sent to gaol for a long term.

We chose to group the divorced and separated together as marriages which had broken down, and together they made up 12 per cent of the total study population or 22 per cent of those ever married. Unfortunately, these could not be compared with official statistics, as those are for divorce or legal separation only.

The data do not reveal whether being adopted adds to the risk of marriage breakdown. It could be that those who marry later will have longer, more stable marriages. Perhaps the study caught the adoptees at the age when the poor results of the early marriages with their greater risk of breakdown were proportionately high. Still, it may be of interest that only seven sets of parents (4 per cent) had been permanently separated or divorced over a much longer period of time. Of course, social attitudes towards divorce have changed and these attitudes are reflected in the Divorce Reform Act, 1969. The rate of divorce has increased year by year (Gibson, 1974, says fiftyfold in the last 60 years). Perhaps the large number of adoptees who had married, compared with only 5 per cent who were cohabiting, may indicate that this group of young people had tried to conform to the standards of morality which most of them almost certainly were taught in these homes. That they were not prepared to continue with the marriage when it had failed may be more characteristic of today's relaxed attitude towards relationships between the sexes and to the emphasis on the right of each individual to find his own happiness.

COMPARISON OF DIRECT AND FOSTER PARENT ADOPTIONS

Length of time to legal adoption
It was expected that the foster children would have been in the family much longer than the others before legal adoption, and this proved to be so. But we were not prepared for the fact that so many of the foster parents had really wanted to adopt and had fostered as a second best, so they were often ready to move right ahead with adoption as soon as the natural mother's consent

could be obtained. In spite of this these adoptions took place much later than the direct adoptions because of the fostering agency's blanket requirement that foster parents must have the child for at least a year before any consideration could be given to their making an application to the court

Table 4.1   *Time in family before adoption order, related to basis on which child was received into family*

	Basis on which child was received into family							
	Adoption only		Fostering with a view to adoption		Fostering only		Total	
	no.	%	no.	%	no.	%	no.	%
Time in family before adoption								
Under 1 year	77	99	6	8	1	7	84	51
1–2 years	1	1	36	50	4	29	41	25
2–5 years	—	—	22	31	3	21	25	15
5 or more years	—	—	8	11	6	43	14	9
Total	78	100	72	100	14	100	164	100

for an Adoption Order, even when the mother had decided sooner to give her consent. As a result of this policy the foster children were very rarely adopted until they had been in the family at least eighteen months to two years, while most of the adoption agency's placements were legalised within three to six months and all but one of them in less than a year (Table 4.1).

Can the fact that so many mothers who had been referred to the fostering agency subsequently decided in a matter of a few months to release their children for adoption be attributed to the agency's policy of encouraging visiting in the foster home to help the mothers decide on the best plan for their children's future? (Just over half did meet the foster parent adopters, mostly on visits to the foster home, and when they found the child had settled, some mothers decided on adoption after one visit). On the other hand, could it indicate that some young mothers (and these mothers were considerably younger as a group than the mothers of the children placed by the adoption agency) had been steered to the fostering agency by their social workers, many of whom at that time did not favour adoption, and the mothers had accepted what was offered without much consideration of alternatives?

Foster parents seem to have received the impression from the fostering agency that adoption was likely to be possible. In a few unfortunate cases a couple who had agreed to foster, when adoption was all they wanted and longed for, were given a foster child whose birth mother had specifically said she would never consider adoption for the baby and in these cases a triangle ensued often lasting many years. Today we would call this a tug of love.

Family place
We had expected that most of the foster children would have older brothers and sisters, but in fact the proportion of foster children who were the first child in the family was almost as high as in the direct adoptions. This probably reflects the foster parents' real wish to adopt. However, in those cases where there were older siblings they were natural-born children of the foster families and likely to be considerably older than the child in the study, in fourteen cases at least ten years older. In the direct adoption cases older siblings usually were adopted children, most often two to five years older, and the child in the study was never more than third in the family, whereas six of the foster children joined their families as the fourth, fifth, or even the sixth child.

Age and socio-economic status of adoptive parents
Like other adopters generally, parents in both our groups tended to be in their thirties when they took these children. Of those mothers who were under 30 or over 40, more than two in three had first had the child either for fostering or for fostering with a view to adoption. Two who took the child only for fostering were over 50 at the time. Actually, in the overall group studied only one in five mothers was in her twenties, the age when most mothers are having their children (Table 4.2).

Three-quarters of the fathers in families who had fostered the children

Table 4.2   *Age of adoptive mother at this placement, related to basis on which child was received into family*

	Basis on which child was received into family					
	Adoption only		Fostering only or with view to adoption		Total	
	no.	%	no.	%	no.	%
Age of adoptive mother						
Under 30	10	*12*	24	*28*	34	*21*
30–39	59	*76*	42	*49*	101	*61*
40 or over	9	*12*	20	*23*	29	*18*
Total	78	*100*	86	*100*	164	*100*

before adopting them were employed as manual or routine clerical workers (social classes III, IV and V in the Registrar General's classification of occupations), while nearly two-thirds of the direct adopters were in professional, semi-professional or managerial work (social classes I and II) (Table 4.3).

Table 4.3   *Social class of adoptive father, related to basis on which child was received into family*

| Social class | Basis on which child was received into family | | | | | | | |
| | Adoption only | | Fostering with a view to adoption | | Fostering only | | Total | |
	no.	%	no.	%	no.	%	no.	%
I	17 }	63	7 }	25	2 }	21	26 }	43
II	32 }		11 }		1 }		44 }	
III	26 }	37	45 }	75	9 }	79	80 }	57
IV	3 }		8 }		2 }		13 }	
V	—	—	1 }		—	—	1 }	
Total	78	*100*	72	*100*	14	*100*	164	*100*

Table 4.4   *Age of child at placement, related to basis on which child was received into family*

| Age of child at placement | Basis on which child was received into family | | | | | |
| | Adoption only | | Fostering only or with a view to adoption | | Total | |
	no.	%	no.	%	no.	%
Under 3 months	48	*62*	14	*16*	62	*38*
3–6 months	18	*23*	41	*48*	59	*36*
6–12 months	9	*11*	20	*23*	29	*18*
12–24 months	3	*4*	6	*7*	9	*5*
24–36 months	—	—	4	*5*	4	*2*
36 months or older	—	—	1	*1*	1	*1*
Total	78	*100*	86	*100*	164	*100*

Adoption is often said to be a middle-class solution to the problem of childlessness and this was even more true at the time these adoptions were being arranged. It is said to be fostering which appeals to working-class mothers who want a young child in the home when their own children are growing up, but it may be that this reflects agency policy more than the wishes of foster parents, since most of our foster parent adopters had always preferred to adopt.

Table 4.5   *Number of prior caretaking arrangements, related to basis on which child was received into family*

	Basis on which child was received into family							
	Adoption only		*Fostering with a view to adoption*		*Fostering only*		*Total*	
	no.	%	no.	%	no.	%	no.	%
Number of prior arrangements								
None – placed from hospital	9	12	—	—	—	—	9	6
One	54	69	7	10	2	14	63	38
Two	11	14	44	61	8	57	63	38
Three	1	1	10	14	2	14	13	8
Four or more	3	4	11	15	1	7	15	9
No information	—	—	—	—	1	8	1	1
Total	78	100	72	100	14	100*	164	100*

* Percentages in tables are rounded to add to 100.

Age at placement and previous living arrangements
Overall, three-quarters of the adoptees had been placed in their families before they were 6 months old and 90 per cent before their first birthday (Table 4.4). The number of caretaking arrangements the children had before this placement is shown in Table 4.5. Children who went to their families specifically for adoption tended to be placed earlier (most often before 3 months) than those who were first fostered by the family (most often at 3 to 6 months) reflecting the fostering agency's policy of receiving all children into its residential nursery before boarding them out with foster parents. This policy was dropped in 1971, and the nursery became a children's day centre, but the procedure was still followed by the agency when the children in the study came into care. So they not only went to their new families later than they otherwise would have, but

they also had this period of residential life, which often lasted longer than intended because of nursery quarantine for various children's diseases. In addition they often spent several days or weeks in hospital if they contracted gastro-enteritis, which at that time was almost endemic wherever babies were cared for in groups.

So we see that there tended to be differences in the experience of the children, their natural parents and their new parents right from the time the children were admitted for placement by one of the two agencies. The foster children tended to be placed later and to have been cared for in a residential nursery for some weeks or months in addition to whatever care arrangements they had already experienced; they more often joined a family where there were older natural-born children and where the parents were more likely to be over 40 or under 30 and of lower socio-economic status than the parents who adopted directly through the adoption society. Birth mothers of the foster children had very often visited in the foster homes before consenting to the adoption, which took place any time up to the age of majority which was then 21. As a matter of agency policy, mothers whose children were placed through the adoption society did not know where their children were; they virtually never met the adopters and all but one of these direct adoptions were completed within one year, most often in less than six months.

PART TWO

---◆---

HOW HAVE THE ADOPTIONS TURNED OUT?

Chapter 5

---◆---

THE PARENTS' OVERALL VIEW

Quite naturally, everyone's first question is 'How did the adoptions turn out?' To assess the overall outcome three separate measures were used. These were the satisfaction of the adoptive parents, the satisfaction of the adopted people and the present life adjustment of these people now in their twenties. The word 'satisfaction' is used here in the sense of meeting expectations, needs or desires, being contented or pleased with, being accepted as adequate. Satisfaction was measured by what adopters and adoptees said in the interviews and the way they said it, both in answer to this particular question and in the overall interview.

Satisfaction on the part of adopters does not necessarily mean that an outsider would consider them satisfactory parents. But taken along with the satisfaction and adjustment of the child, it is a useful measure of adoption outcome as well as being of interest in its own right. Much of the information in adoption research has come from parents' description of their children, which surely reflects their own satisfaction or disappointment, and a few follow-up studies have given special consideration to the parents' satisfaction (Witmer et al., 1963; Kadushin, 1970; Tizard, 1977). This chapter will consider the satisfaction of adoptive parents in the project, the next chapter will deal with the satisfaction of the adopted people and that will be followed by a chapter on their present adult adjustment.

Some children are, of course, much easier to love than others, and each child brings his own temperament and brief experience of life with him when he enters a new family. The whole family configuration changes when a new person, even a very tiny one, enters it; each person now reacts to all the others in a somewhat different way and each contributes something to the emotional climate of the home. So, while parental influence on the child is very great, the child's individuality is not without its effect upon the parents and upon their interaction with him. We have all known parents who respond differently to each of their children and there is evidence that children's individual differences may be crucial in determining how parents respond to them (Rutter, 1970).

OVERALL OUTCOME

'She is just our daughter, satisfactory in every way'

The 160 sets of adopters who were interviewed were now in their fifties, sixties and even seventies, and in these interviews they were looking back over the last 20-odd years. For 85 per cent of them (136 families) the adoption of the children in the study had been a satisfying experience. These include 105 (66 per cent) who were really enthusiastic, who had found it a very satisfying and richly rewarding experience and who considered the adoption an unqualified success. They also include 31 (19 per cent) who assessed their experience as reasonably satisfactory, but not entirely so (Table 5.1).

Table 5.1   *Adoptive parents' overall experience with child*

	No. of families	%	
Experience			
Very satisfactory	105	*66* }	*85*
Reasonably satisfactory	31	*19* }	
Mainly unsatisfactory	14	*9* }	*14*
Very unsatisfactory	8	*5* }	
Incompatible responses from mother and father	2	*1*	
Total	160*	*100*	

* Although the total number of cases involved in the project was 164, tables showing information from parent interviews are necessarily based on 160, as only 160 sets of parents participated. In the other four families only the adoptee could be interviewed.

Many parents said that the child had brought them much happiness and they had no regrets. As one father said: 'It went like a bomb.' Others thought the adoption was 'totally satisfying'; it had made their lives and was the best thing they had ever done. A father spoke of his boy as all a man could want in a son. Other parents said they had enjoyed a happy family life with a lovable child and now there were the grandchildren. The Brown family said they had had a happy time with their son; he was an easy and conforming child who took to their ways readily and was very satisfactory in every way. A number of parents with only this one child had found the experience so rewarding that they deeply regretted not having a larger adopted family. Perhaps any earlier reservations about a larger family had been put aside now that things had turned out well.

In rating their experience as satisfying, parents were not necessarily saying there had been no problems. The study tends to confirm that for certain adoptive parents something much less than an ideal or problem-free situation can prove satisfying over the years if the difficulties have some compensations. Even acute anxiety, serious disappointment or severe practical problems can be contained. One parent said: 'We never looked upon him as adopted. He has always just been ours; we always hoped we could adopt him but always thought of him as ours anyway.' This family were finally able to adopt their foster child legally after seven years. Several others who had fostered their child first said everything about the experience was fine except the long period of nerve-racking uncertainty before they were able to legally adopt the youngster they had come to love as their own.

A father now 75 and widowed said convincingly that it had been a happy experience in spite of the daughter being a slow learner and 'mildly epileptic'. It was his opinion that nearly all good things in life have some cost one way or another and he and his wife had never regretted taking this child.

A mother said of her son, who had a serious heart condition when placed with her as a foster child: 'I was told he was not a perfect baby but I said I would foster him since he needed a home, and we later adopted him and are very glad we did.' Another kind and homely family had taken a little boy who today would have been labelled a battered child, and they had found great satisfaction in seeing him grow into a less insecure child whom they loved as their own, although he had never been able to achieve much in school. The warm and loving mother of another boy, who was so backward that the agency delayed the legal adoption for several years, said the boy was just as a natural son, kind, honest, hard-working, helpful and 'you couldn't ask for a better son'.

Mr Smith spoke with satisfaction about how he had coped with bringing up his son after the adoptive mother died, and in another case it was the mother who was widowed and had found it hard bringing up a son alone but it had given her great satisfaction. Parents of a girl who had been dreadfully difficult in adolescence, rejecting all the family's values, rated the overall experience as satisfying and worthwhile because it had all turned out well. When we saw them, the daughter had married a young man they thoroughly approved of and they were once again a closely knit, happy family.

Asked what they liked most in their son or daughter, parents most often mentioned that the young person was kind, thoughtful or considerate. Sometimes they said with approval 'He would do anything for anyone', but more often they were pleased because as an adult he was now kind and thoughtful to them. Next most often mentioned was the adoptee's disposition; he was good-natured and cheerful, an open person, fun to be with. That the adoptee was affectionate and loving towards them was very important. Being generous, making friends easily and getting along well with people were traits which were often mentioned. Asked what they liked least about the child, many of the satisfied adopters could not think of anything. Others could think of only something very minor which had been a passing phase in the process of growing up – long hair at university, untidy dress, loud pop music or refusal to help in the house.

'He is just an entirely different kind of animal'
The 14 per cent of parents who had *not* found their overall experience with the adopted child satisfying was made up of 22 families. Fourteen of these had found the experience disappointing on the whole, though not entirely so, but eight described the experience as very unsatisfactory and disappointing. In the two remaining families, which have not been included here in either the satisfied or dissatisfied groups, the parents thoroughly disagreed, one having found it satisfactory and the other not at all so.

It is surely noteworthy that in every one of the eight cases of real parental dissatisfaction the child concerned was a boy. Yet it is difficult to assess the meaning of this finding, as overall the sex of the adoptees evidently had little or nothing to do with parental satisfaction. The satisfied group of 136 adoptive families included 84 per cent of those with a son in the study and 87 per cent of those with a daughter, and sons and daughters were spoken of with equal warmth and concern. However, boys in the general population are known to be more prone than girls to problems of health, development or behaviour and several other studies have shown this to be true of adopted children (Witmer *et al.*, 1963; Jaffee and Fanshel, 1970; Bohman, 1970; Seglow *et al.*, 1972).

Among the small group of 22 families with a largely unsatisfactory or very unsatisfactory experience were two where the son in the study was permanently hospitalised, one with very severe epilepsy and the other severely subnormal, and two other families in which a daughter was mentally handicapped (one educationally subnormal and with limited sight and the other severely subnormal and subject to periods of mental illness as well). Probably very few parents would have found their experience really satisfying with these four children who developed such serious handicaps, and three of these families certainly had made the best of the situation. The other 18 families disliked their child's personality for one reason or another, and most of these believed this was because the child was not born to them and they were unable to mould him or her to their ways. There were very few instances of parents accepting responsibiity for an undesirable outcome. When things worked out badly it probably reinforced the feelings of self-doubt that adopters so often entertain about themselves as parents, but some placements may simply have been from the beginning what Kadushin and Seidl (1971) have called 'failing combinations'. Of course, parents of natural-born children, too, find it very unpleasant to feel they have failed with their children.

Parents of at least three children in the study viewed them in such a detached way that they seemed to be describing a clinical specimen. The father in one of these families felt that a prediction he had made when they decided to adopt had been shown to be correct, that an adopted child would never be as their own and would not amount to much. A father with three adopted sons was disappointed that none of them was as totally masculine as he would have liked and he had now become largely indifferent to them. Another father said sadly: 'There was always a barrier.' Although this failed adoption was greatly complicated by the adoptive mother's extreme rigidity and the breakdown of the marriage, the father's real dissatisfaction with it was because he was never able to establish the real father–son relationship he longed for. He tended to blame this on the son, while showing little awareness of the poor family situation in which the boy had developed the emotional problems and personality traits which the father later could not tolerate.

One case provided a striking example of a self-fulfilling prophecy and there had never been any real chance of a happy outcome. It would be inappropriate here to try to say what psychological mechanisms were at work that drove this couple to add to the natural children in their family by adopting an illegitimate baby, when they were firmly convinced that being born illegitimate amounted to a curse which would make a normal life impossible and that being adopted cast an evil shadow over any child's future. They had never been hesitant in letting the child know of their forebodings and he had left home at an early age and had not let them know his whereabouts. They were sure that he had been in trouble and they felt that all their worst fears had been well-founded.

In another family a professional man felt dissatisfied with the adoption because his relationship with his son was not close and rewarding. This father was greatly disappointed because the boy had failed to carry on the family tradition for excellence in sport, and he had blinded himself to the fact that the boy was intellectually quite brilliant and was now making good use of his fine mind in another profession.

Two families had never had any really strong motivation to adopt the foster child in their home and it was not very clear why they had done so. In one of these two families the child had been taken to please the whim of a much older natural-born child who had seen an advertisement for foster homes for babies. The child was returned to the agency twice, first as a baby and later as a toddler. The foster mother said she had been made to feel 'wicked' when she returned the baby to the agency, so after a few weeks she asked to take him back. The second time she returned him saying he was 'out of control', but after a bit she agreed to try again after the agency had arranged day nursery care so she could take part-time employment. Somewhat later, the family legally adopted this child, the mother explaining this by saying that they had got rather attached to him. Not surprisingly, this adoption did not work out well from the standpoint of anyone concerned and the child was later taken into care of the local authority at the request of the adopters, when he was again said to be out of control.

Asked what they liked about their child, even those children who were otherwise very unsatisfactory to their parents were often described as being generous with cards and gifts at the appropriate times. This seemed to mean a great deal to some otherwise unhappy parents, who perhaps interpreted this as a residue of caring in a relationship which had become largely negative, or perhaps they saw it as evidence that the child still held fast to at least a few of the customs of the culture in which they had brought him up.

When asked what they liked least about their child, it was the child's poor academic showing or his lack of interest in school which was most often mentioned (27 cases), followed by 13 cases in which the child was said to have no ambition or no staying power to achieve any skill. (Even among the satisfied parents some complained about the child's poor school record, though they tended to discount this in cases where the adoptee was now doing well in a career even without the usual educational qualifications.) Lack of school effort or achievement and lack of ambition to make something of themselves, these seemed to be the two points, and they were obviously closely related, on which parents and children most often had differing values. When failure to share the family's values extended to other areas of life, as well as to education and ambition to achieve, parents were always unhappy and dissatisfied, and complained that the child had not responded to 'moulding'.

A few mentioned that they found the child, now a young adult, selfish or superficial, restless or materialistic. One girl had been 'boy crazy'; two boys were described as 'cowardly' because they tended not to face up to problems. Other traits which parents found most distasteful included being ungrateful, delinquent or promiscuous, self-willed or quick-tempered. Two or three parents were critical of a son's smoking or drinking. One father, a professional man, characterised as a plodder a son who is now in the same profession. Another family were critical of a boy not bright enough to carry on the father's small business, and still another mentioned their disturbed boy's threats of violence towards them when frustrated.

Moulding. The word 'mould' was used over and over again by these people who had parented children not born to them. Some who were happy with the adoption used the word saying how easily the child had moulded to their ways and become one of the family. But it could be said of most of the little group of dissatisfied adopters that they had felt urgently the need to mould the child to their ways, but believed they had failed in this because the pull of some unknown genetic factors had been too strong. They had tried to prevent the child from developing in his own way, and had worked harder and harder to squeeze him into the imagined likeness of the ideal child who should have been born to them, but the harder they worked the more the child resisted their efforts. A boy said with considerable self-awareness that his rebellion (and there was a great deal of rebellion and acting out on his part) was for a chance to grow up and be himself. One adoptive father said of his son: 'He was a lovely little boy until he began to spread his wings.' A constant struggle to mould this boy had been completely unsuccessful and was, in fact, still going on, as shown by the fact that the father told us the son was welcome in the parental home only if he did not do anything to irritate him.

Fathers seemed to come into conflict with adopted children, usually sons, much more often than mothers, especially in this matter of moulding a child to their ways. It often showed up in families where the mother had died or the parents had been divorced. Where it occurred in families still intact, the mother usually agreed, at least tacitly, with the father's views, and the adoption had in any case been unsatisfactory because of the conflict between father and son. More than 20 years ago, when these children were being placed, the wishes and personality of the prospective adoptive father were not often considered when applications were being assessed, at least in the two agencies studied, and it may be that some male adopters either had grave doubts about the venture from the beginning or very little idea of how adoption would be different from having a natural-born child.

As might be predicted, strong-willed children with 'moulding' parents often developed personalities which freed them from the parental grip but did not make it easy for them to get on with their friends or workmates, their spouses or children, and some of them were found later among the less well-adjusted young adults in the study.

Table 5.2   *Parents' overall experience with child, related to social class of adoptive father*

	Social class of adoptive father										
	Social class I		Social class II		Social class III		Social class IV		Social class V		Total	
	no.	%	no.	%	no.	%	no.	%	no.	%	no.	%
Parents' experience												
Satisfactory	22	88	37	86	66	84	11	85	—	—	136	85
Unsatisfactory	3	12	4	9	13	16	2	15	—	—	22	14
Incompatible responses	—	—	2	5	—	—	—	—	—	—	2	1
Total	25	100	43	100	79	100	13	100	—	—	160	100

FACTORS ASSOCIATED WITH PARENTAL SATISFACTION

Age and social class of adopters
Age and social class did not seem to be important factors in parental

satisfaction with adoption. In the great majority of cases, regardless of socio-economic status adoption had proved over the years to be an acceptable way of having children (Table 5.2). The age of the adoptive mother showed only a weak relationship and that of the father apparently none at all.

Early experience with the child
Although some children at placement had been quite different from the adoptive parents' mental image of the child they had hoped to make their own (different in age, sex, appearance, etc.), no apparent relationship was found between this and the parents' overall satisfaction with the adoption. However, satisfaction *was* related to how quickly and easily the child settled into their home. Only one in ten who now assessed their experience as satisfying had a child who had taken a long time to settle, while one in three of the dissatisfied parents had such a child. Sometimes the process had taken months or even years, and indeed in four cases the adopters felt the child had never really settled. Adopters as well as children had sometimes found adjustment to the placement difficult. Indeed, in one case already mentioned in which the child was returned twice to the agency before legal adoption, parents indicated they *never* had adjusted to parenting the child, and in eight additional cases one of the parents (four fathers and four mothers) had never made the adjustment to that role. It is not surprising that the four adoptees mentioned above, who had never settled, were in these families where one or both adoptive parents had never adjusted to parenting them.

Adopters' early doubts about the child or about themselves as his parents were recorded at the time in only 11 cases, but during the research interview 38 families acknowledged that doubts or uncertainties had in fact troubled them more than 20 years before. One in every two of those assessing their experience of adoption as unsatisfactory now said there had been early doubts, while this was true of only one in five of the satisfied. Perhaps some agency workers, in their eagerness that all should go well, had not always recognised or recorded the adopters' uncertainties. In the early contacts adopters may not have been encouraged to express any doubts or they may have been fearful of their agency's reaction, since agencies are seen as powerful and adopters are well known to be very vulnerable until they have been able to complete the legal adoption. Then, too, a few families may later have rationalised their growing discontent with the adoption by believing they had always thought it might turn out this way.

Some parents were critical of the way they were introduced to the child and this first meeting was still a very vivid memory and occasionally a traumatic one. In those days adopters, or the adoptive mother alone, were summoned to come to an agency office or nursery to see the child who had been selected for them and they were expected to be prepared to take him home immediately if they wanted him.

An adoptive mother spoke of having to make a decision 'when you walk into the room under pressure not to say "No" or you go to the end of the queue'. Several criticised being offered a choice of two or three children in a residential nursery or they remembered noticing other children in the nursery who seemed a better choice than the one they were offered.

A father who had accompanied his wife to a residential nursery to see the baby the agency was offering them for fostering with a view to adoption said he felt he was in a showroom being shown around by a saleswoman (the matron). He said: 'Choosing a second-hand car is bad enough, but going into a Home and choosing a baby is a hundred times worse – imagine looking at babies and saying, "I don't want that one, I don't want that one"; it's a horrible situation and something I wouldn't want to do again.' This man went on to tell the interviewer that he and his wife were shown a very dark, foreign-looking baby and the matron seemed to be trying to talk them into having that one, but when they refused she showed them another, also very dark, and they did not feel right about that baby either, so he said: 'No – after all it's important; it's for a lifetime.' Then they spied a baby with a mass of very fair hair. The man said: 'All my relatives had very fair hair when they were little, so I told the matron that was the one we wanted, and we felt he was one of us already because of his mop of fair hair.' Unfortunately, the hair did not prove a very sound indicator of affinity, as the parents tended to emphasise the boy's difference from them when the adoption did not go well. However, the unpleasant scene in the nursery was still crystal clear in this father's mind.

More often when a child was first taken for fostering only the foster/adoptive mother had so much as seen the child until he was in the home. As prospective fathers were seldom interviewed when the home was being assessed and were not often present at the placement, they often had little, if any, part in the venture until a child was settling into the family. One woman had deliberately kept her husband ignorant of her plan to foster a child with a view to adoption until the child was actually in the home. There must have been many parents who had second thoughts about what they had undertaken!

Family place and age at placement
Parents often felt quite differently towards one child from the way they felt towards the others. Sometimes the child in the study was one they were enthusiastic about, but in some other families he was the odd man out and parents spoke disparagingly of him while extolling the virtues of another child, usually also adopted. However, satisfaction or discontent with a child in the study did not seem to be associated with family place except that in the six cases where this child was the fourth, fifth, or sixth child the adoptive parents were in every case well satisfied. Nor did the age of the child when placed with the family show any apparent association with parental satisfaction, although it should be remembered that more than nine out of

ten of these children were under 1 year old at placement and the eldest was a boy of 4. There was no indication that dissatisfaction was related to later placement, and in fact the children of all the eight most dissatisfied adopters had been placed before they were 1 year old.

Legalisation

In more than 75 per cent of the families legal adoption was completed within two years and usually during the first year when it was a direct adoption. Among children taken only with the intention of fostering, legal adoption often did not occur until much later, but this did not seem to affect the satisfaction parents felt in the adoption (Table 5.3). Even though great

Table 5.3 *Adoptive parents' overall experience with this child, related to length of time to adoption order*

	Length of time to adoption order									
	Less than one year		1–2 years		2–5 years		5 or more years		Total	
	no.	%	no.	%	no.	%	no.	%	no.	%
Parents' overall experience										
Satisfactory	71	86	35	85	19	79	11	92	136	85
Unsatisfactory	11	13	5	12	5	21	1	8	22	14
Incompatible responses	1	1	1	3	—	—	—	—	2	1
Total	83	100	41	100	24	100	12	100	160	100

anxiety had been created by repeated delays in legalising the adoption, and this had caused much insecurity and unhappiness for parents and children, yet these people usually felt that the overall experience with the child had been rewarding and worthwhile. Of the 12 families who waited longest (five years or more before an adoption order was granted), all but one assessed their overall experience as satisfactory. We do know a family, mentioned earlier, who refused to take part in the study (and are therefore not included in these figures) because they could not bear to open up the subject of the adoption, as the years of waiting for legalisation had been so painful and the resentment against the agency so great. There is also some reason to think that there may have been other foster parents, not included in this study because they never adopted a foster child in their home, who would have wished to adopt the child but were put off by the delays and possibly sometimes by the loss of boarding-out fees to which they had become accustomed over the years.

Basis of placement
One of the central questions underlying the whole project was whether adopting one's foster child is likely to be as satisfactory and rewarding as adopting a child directly from an adoption agency. The results show no apparent difference in the proportion of satisfied parents among those who had taken a child directly for adoption and those who had first fostered him. However, within the fostering group there was a noticeable difference in the degree of satisfaction or dissatisfaction between the 14 'true' foster parents and the much larger number who had fostered with a view to adoption. The 'true' foster parents were too few in number for any conclusions to be drawn, but the results may be of interest nevertheless. Those 'true' foster parents who were satisfied with the experience were evenly divided between parents who were very satisfied and those who were only moderately so, whereas when the parents who had adopted the child directly or had fostered with a view to adoption were satisfied, they were much more often very satisfied and enthusiastic. Only two 'true' foster parents rated their experience as unsatisfactory, but these had found it very unsatisfactory indeed (Table 5.4).

Table 5.4   *Parents' overall experience with child, related to basis on which child was received into family*

	Basis on which child was received into family							
	Adoption only		Fostering with a view		Fostering only		Total	
	no.	%	no.	%	no.	%	no.	%
Parents' experience								
Very satisfactory	50	⌐65	49	⌐71	6	⌐43	105	⌐66
		86⟨		84⟨		86⟨		85⟨
Reasonably satisfactory	16	⌊21	9	⌊13	6	⌊43	31	⌊19
Mainly unsatisfactory	8	10	6	9	—	—	14	9
Very unsatisfactory	2	3	4	6	2	14	8	5
Incompatible responses	1	1	1	1	—	—	2	1
Total	77	100	69	100	14	100	160	100

Although those who had fostered first were in general nearly as satisfied as the direct adopters, this did not mean that they were in favour of this method of achieving their family. An overwhelming majority of the parents in the study made it very clear that they saw no advantage in fostering first, and indeed saw many serious disadvantages in taking the child first on this basis. Only 14 (9 per cent) of the 160 parents interviewed in the project saw any advantage at all in fostering the child first and 5 of these 14 felt it also had disadvantages. The main advantages, of course, were that one had time to be sure the child was 'all right' and that the child and family were suited to each other. Even the few who felt these were important usually recommended a much shorter period of fostering than they themselves had experienced, and they nearly always qualified their statement by adding the proviso that they would have to be assured that they definitely would be able to adopt the child at some time, an assurance an agency alone could not give.

None of the parents who had adopted the child directly through the adoption agency wished they had fostered the child first or saw any advantage in doing so. They were willing to take the risk of the child not being 'all right' rather than to foster him first to find out about this. Most of them said they never would have fostered first because fostering was too insecure. Their view of fostering was that 'it is neither here nor there, it is insecure for everyone concerned', and they did not want to have anything to do with it. They spoke of being anxious enough during the few months until these direct adoptions were legalised; they would not have been prepared to go through a period of fostering which would have meant a longer experience of fear and uncertainty. A woman who had adopted directly and was able to complete the adoption in the minimum time under the law said: 'Even so, I shook all the way to the court fearing the natural mother might turn up and take the baby.'

All the adoptive parents who had procured their child through the fostering agency, except the 14 already mentioned, thought fostering the child first had been a disadvantage. Many recalled the difficulties and delays surrounding the legal process of adopting their foster child and said they could never go through it again. As we have already seen, many had fostered the child only as a step necessary for them in the adoption process. They often said they would have adopted directly through an adoption agency if they had not been ineligible because of adoption agency regulations on the age of adopters and the number of their natural-born children. They would not have taken the child first on a fostering basis if they could have done it in any other way.

As it was, these people had made a full commitment to the child right from the start. They had taken him with a view to adoption in spite of the fact that they had applied to a fostering agency which was not registered to place children for adoption, and in face of the fact that the child's natural mother usually had not been expected to release her child for adoption. It is not surprising therefore that before they could reach their goal, they usually had to cope with a series of delays and postponed decisions which seemed to take even longer than they actually did. What is striking is the degree of anguish they sometimes experienced and the way in which the anxiety evidently affected not only the would-be adopters but the natural parents and the children too. The interviews provided many examples of what has been termed 'the corrosive impact of uncertainty'.

In these cases of fostering with a view to adoption the natural mothers had been encouraged to 'take a breathing space' in which to consider the pros and cons of bringing up the babies themselves or relinquishing them for adoption, but during the breathing space they seem to have been given very little help in coming to a decision. They continued to waver, sometimes for years or in a few cases until a child was nearly grown up, before deciding to relinquish him for adoption by the foster parents. The stress of this long-drawn-out decision on the mother and her family must have been very great, and meanwhile the foster parents lived with uncertainty and a constant fear that she would one day reclaim the child they had come to love as their own. Foster children, too, lived with this uncertainty about their status and found it hard to accept that their surnames were different and that an agency instead of parents had control over various important aspects of their lives.

Often foster parents had understood from the agency representative that the child they were taking would be available to them for adoption after one year as a foster child in their home, but when it did not work out as quickly or simply as that they felt they had been subjected to all the natural mother's uncertainties. One adopter said the baby's mother had second thoughts after the placement and 'every time she visited she turned the knife'. As one mother expressed it: 'There is too much strain in fostering the child first. I don't ever want to live through those two years again. We lived on the edge of a precipice.' Another family said the worry and anxiety over this was worse than anything else that had ever happened to them and they believed that the child, who was nervous and clinging, had sensed their distress.

More than one mother spoke of being afraid to answer a knock at the door or said she had been worried that the birth mother might snatch the sleeping baby from the pram in front of the house. In a case where it 'took five years to get the mother's consent' a foster/adoptive mother said they were 'five years of nerve-racking worry', fearing every day the postman would bring a letter saying they must return the child. A few had already had a child reclaimed before they took this one, so they were even more anxious than most to get the natural mother's consent and legalise the adoption quickly. A woman with two natural-born children said: 'Never foster if you want to adopt. It was awfully hard having my sons by birth, but adopting them was much harder.' Another family had found the mother's visiting and her uncertainty about giving her consent very anxiety-provoking and to this day they still worry that she will turn up.

Some people who had fostered when they really wanted to adopt had felt uncomfortable about the fostering fees. Some even sent the fees back to the agency after the adoption had been completed, and one father had written in his diary 'Received payment from Pharaoh for looking after Moses'.

In spite of the difficulties so many of these parents recalled around the adoption, most spoke well of their individual social worker and not all who had encountered difficulties were bitter towards the fostering agency. Perhaps seeing a mother who was reluctant and uncertain about giving up all claim to her child made some adopters feel they must suffer equally with her in order to feel they had any right to parent that child.

Though often a cause for anxiety, the contact with the mother could also be seen as a definite benefit, and there were two families who gave the chance to know the natural mother as the advantage they saw in fostering first. These had wanted more information from her and had felt more fully entitled to the child because they had liked the mother and were able to identify with her.

A father's reason for favouring a period of fostering was the opportunity it had given him to work through his own conflicting feelings about adoption, and for him this opportunity outweighed the anxieties of the fostering period. Today we would hope that conflicting feelings would be worked through with the agency before a child was placed.

Whereas most people wanted to achieve legal adoption as soon as possible, a few had been glad of a chance to delay it. One family said fostering first was an advantage because it gave them a chance to know the child and they knew adoption was 'not something to be rushed into'. This was a family who did not legally adopt their foster son until late adolescence. Although they were not really short of money, the adoptive mother tended to be anxious about money, so it may be that reluctance to lose the income from fostering fees was a strong contributing factor in the delay.

Problems in growing up

Any health or developmental problems the children had before coming to these families, or during the period before legal adoption, had not affected parental satisfaction. Seven children had been thought very early on by the agency, or by the adopters, to be slow in their development, but only four of these particular children continued to develop in this way and six of the seven had parents who were satisfied. Presumably these adopters had proceeded with the adoption with their eyes open, so there was none of the disappointment that was engendered when, as in some other cases, a handicapping condition developed later. (This will be discussed in detail in Chapter 11.)

Behaviour problems were very seldom mentioned in the case files, that is, before the legal adoption, as most of the children were still very young and adopters would in any case have been fearful that mentioning any problems they were having with the child might result in the agency withdrawing him from their care. But behaviour or personality problems while the child was growing up in the family after legal adoption were a different matter and the parents of these children were less often satisfied with the adoption than were those who reported no such problems. Of course it is impossible at this stage to know whether some element of rejection, or at least lack of full commitment and affection, may have caused some of the behaviour problems or personality traits which the parents subsequently complained about. In this regard it is interesting that the families most often rating their overall experience as satisfactory were those where both parents had been deeply involved with the child over the years, and if there were other children the parents had been equally involved with them too.

In the matter of discipline most parents tended to feel they had exerted moderate or even minimal control over the child, but of the eight parents who were very dissatisfied five thought they had been inconsistent and three believed they had been strict. Parents often said they had been less strict than their own parents and that their circumstances had allowed them to provide their children with more material things than they themselves had been given.

Similarity of child and adoptive parents
The clearest link between parental satisfaction and any one factor which was explored was the adoptive parents' perception of the child as being similar to them in some way, such as appearance, general intelligence, temperament, mannerisms, talents or skills (Table 5.5).

Table 5.5 *Adoptive parents' overall experience with child, related to their perception of the child as like them*

	Adoptive parents' feeling of likeness to child								
	Like		Unlike		Incompat-ible responses		Not covered		Total	
	no.	%	no.	%	no.	%	no.	%	no.	%
Parents' experience										
Satisfactory	94	97	33	62	1	100	8	89	136	85
Unsatisfactory	2	2	19	36	—	—	1	11	22	14
Incompatible responses	1	1	1	2	—	—	—	—	2	1
Total	97	100	53	100	1	100	9	100	160	100

A few parents who had felt their adopted child was very different from them had let it create a barrier between them but others had not. A doting mother said of her son, 'There has always been something different about him; he is not working class', but this working-class family nevertheless always felt the son 'belonged'. In another family the daughter was described as 'classy'. Several parents saw their child as less bright and less academic than themselves, and there were at least three bright and well-educated adoptees who were seen as different and not very bright by parents who were even more intellectual. Then of course there were those who disapproved so much of their child's temperament, life-style or lack of achievement, or in one case his illegitimacy, that they could only see the adoptee as entirely different from themselves.

Nearly all those who thought the child was like them were satisfied with the adoption, but less than two-thirds were satisfied when the child was seen as different. Putting it another way, we see that only two of the twenty-two pairs of dissatisfied adopters saw the child as somewhat like them. The cause and effect relationship is not known but there certainly is an association. Of course, it is easier for parents to identify a child with themselves when their experience with him is satisfactory; but is not the experience with him more likely to be satisfactory if the child is enough like the adoptive parents to be easily understood and empathised with? At any rate it is evident that the adopters were pleased at being able to see some likeness to themselves in their child – a very normal parental pleasure.

These findings are interesting in view of the controversy over 'matching' which has been going on in social work circles for some years. The implications for practice will be considered in the final chapter.

Relationship with the agency
As we have seen, most adoptive parents felt rather warmly towards their agency social worker. Only one in four felt the placement agency could have been more helpful to them at some time. Half the dissatisfied parents now felt this but only one-fifth of the satisfied. Some people wished for more medical information or for the child's birth certificate. Former foster parents felt their agency could have given them more support in achieving the legalisation. They believed the agency had not really wanted them to adopt and had put obstacles in their way or at least had left the foster parents themselves to contact the birth mother and get her consent. (At that time the fostering agency was not registered to place children for adoption and believed it would be illegal to enter into the negotiations, so foster parents wishing to adopt and approved by the agency were given the birth mother's address and left to contact her for her consent.)

Two or three families felt their agency could have done a better job of 'matching' a child to their family, especially one mother who thought the agency should have known that a child from a working-class background would never fit into their upper-middle-class family. A few had found that friends and relatives had given conflicting advice and that they would have benefited from some instruction in baby care – how to handle feeding problems or a fretful baby, or what to do about excessive crying or poor sleeping habits. Another family felt they should have had more help before placement in order to realise the full implications of what they were taking on, since adopters are 'stuck with their decision for 20 years'.

In a few cases there appeared to be a discrepancy between the declared policy of the agency and the attitudes of the staff. In an example of this the adoptive parents were very bitter because they felt the agency had not been honest with them. This family had fostered the child only in order to adopt and they had understood that the mother was offering the baby for adoption. Some months later they learned that the mother had never planned to release the child and, although she eventually did so, a struggle ensued over many months before the adoption could be completed. The adoptive mother had been terribly upset by this and later problems were attributed to this unhappy beginning.

A few parents saw the possibility of the agency being helpful to their children much later if they wanted more information about their natural parents or just wanted to talk about their background or visit the agency to see 'where they came from'. Some of these were parents who had not been able to discuss background with their children and wondered if the agency might have done it for them.

In this chapter we have seen that most, but not all, of the adoptions had worked out well from the viewpoint of the adoptive parents, and they looked back on the experience of the last 20-odd years with a great deal of pleasure and satisfaction.

Chapter 6

———◆———

THE ADOPTED PEOPLE'S OVERALL VIEW

We went to the adopted people themselves to learn about adoption from the receiving end, as they were the only ones who could say what growing up adopted had really been like for them. We wanted to be able to compare their experiences and feelings with those of their parents and to find out what factors seemed most closely linked with satisfaction – or lack of it.

The project staff wondered whether things that social workers thought would be important to a child had proved to be so, for instance, adoptive parents' age or social class, their attitude to heredity and background, and whether they also had children born to them. It was thought that being fostered for several years before adoption might have affected the satisfaction of the children, so it would be interesting to know how they felt about it now that they were adults. In all the interviews it was planned to continue testing the relevance and validity of theories which other researchers had raised and which we had started to explore during discussions with the adopters. This chapter considers how satisfying the young people had found their overall adoption experience and provides some general information about the factors associated with this. Issues which proved particularly important or interesting are picked up again for fuller discussion in subsequent chapters.

The project staff was able to interview 105 of the adult adoptees, 59 men and 46 women. Contrary to the general belief that follow-up studies are likely to involve a larger number of 'successful' than 'unsuccessful' adoptions, and if successful and satisfactory are considered to be analogous, somewhat the reverse appears to have been the case here. Rather to our surprise, satisfied adopters were somewhat less often willing for their son or daughter to take part in the research (69 per cent willing) than were the parents who had suffered a disappointing experience (77 per cent willing), but the difference was not statistically significant. In addition more adoptees from satisfied families refused an interview for themselves or were not available. Parents who felt satisfied with the adoption were often very protective of their children as well as fearful of doing anything to disturb the *status quo* in the family. One adoptive mother put it very plainly when she said that it might upset her happily married daughter and make her want to find her first mother and not want the adopters any more.

Most adoptees talked less freely than their parents and seemed to have less to say. They often thought adoption was so natural that they did not know what to say about it as they had no other experience with which to compare it. They were protective of their adoptive parents and showed real understanding of the panic their parents felt in discussing adoption with them. They were very loyal and often did not criticise their parents even when their own experience in the family had been unhappy. They were also more ready than their parents to take the blame for problems.

ADOPTION AS A LIFE EXPERIENCE

'I have no problems about being adopted; it has always been accepted, not talked about, just accepted, that's all.'

'It hangs like a great black cloud over everything and overshadows everything else.'

Four out of five of the adoptees who were interviewed were satisfied with their experience of adoption. Those who assessed their experience as more or less evenly balanced have been counted here among the dissatisfied, since they had not felt able to say it had been satisfactory and other things they said in the interview led us to believe they were not really satisfied (Table 6.1). Most of the adoptees whose parents had thought they were happy in their adoption really were, but so were half of those the parents were uncertain about or had thought were dissatisfied. There were seven adoptees who were satisfied even though their parents were not, and two of these in particular seemed oblivious of their parents' keen disappointment in them. There were also 12 adoptees who were not happy with their adoption though the parents were satisfied with them. So, in all, there was disagreement about how the adoption had turned out in 19 of the cases where both children and parents were interviewed.

Table 6.1   *Adoptees' satisfaction with their experience of growing up adopted*

Adoptees' experience	no.		%	
Very satisfactory	60 }	83	58 }	80
Reasonably satisfactory	23 }		22 }	
Mainly unsatisfactory	18 }	21	17 }	20
Very unsatisfactory	3 }		3 }	
Total	104*		100	

* Figures exclude one who could not be questioned on his experience of adoption.

Only three adoptees were really dissatisfied, although in view of the experience of some others it would not have been surprising if a few more had assessed it this way. Of the three who were very unhappy in their adoption, one was a young woman who had been placed in a very busy and incredibly class-conscious family, who attributed everything, good or bad, to heredity. The girl was given good physical care and educational and material advantages in an upper-middle-class home, but she felt unloved and was convinced that her family had never really wanted children and had adopted only because it was the socially acceptable thing to do. She felt her parents were too old and rigid to adopt and had expected the children to be perfect.

The second very dissatisfied adoptee had been a bright but very difficult and strong-willed lad placed with an unsophisticated family, where the father appears to have played a weak role, and the mother in spite of much effort was unable to understand or control the boy's behaviour. He said that even as a young child he had felt rejected and 'on the outside looking in'. He now had nothing but criticism for these parents, although he consciously tried to accept them. The third was John, a man who felt his adoption had been a disaster. Certainly it had been sad and difficult for all concerned. He was brought up in a very simple family where an earlier and much-loved baby had been reclaimed by its birth mother only weeks before this son joined the family. Apparently, the adoptive mother had not been able to work through her grief at the time, as nearly 25 years later at the research interview she wept bitterly for her lost baby. The son said he had always been compared unfavourably with the reclaimed child and furthermore had sometimes been subjected to 'beatings' by his father. Not surprisingly, he had soon given up trying to please and had fallen in with a group of delinquents. Corporal punishment was not unusual at that time, and in interviewing the father we felt he was genuinely fond of the son and had done what he thought was best for him.

Almost none of the adoptees had envisaged growing up in any other family, whether natural, foster or adoptive, but quite a few offered the opinion that they felt lucky to have been chosen and to have avoided what most of them saw as the alternative, that is, growing up in a children's home.

Some people had given surprisingly little thought to the subject of their adoption or else they were denying whatever feelings they had about it, but the project's experienced interviewers did not often assess it as denial. These people could only say they had always known they were adopted and they had not been bothered by it. Typical was a young woman who said she had always felt these were her parents, as they had made her feel loved and wanted, and one who said she had never really thought about being adopted and did not feel different from anyone else. Another said she never thinks about it until the subject is raised by someone else. A young man said his life had been uneventful and probably not very different from what it would have been in the family he was born to. The idea of adoption never worried him. Another young man said it would never occur to him to think of not belonging to his family, and still another said: 'They treated me well and I was happy with them. Everything has gone fine for me so there is nothing more to say. I am not bothered about my background – Mum and Dad are my parents and that's that.'

Others who had thought more about their adoption were able to say more about how it felt. Two or three people, because they were adopted, had always felt a good deal of responsibility not to do anything that would hurt their parents, but two others took a different view of this, saying they were sure they had fulfilled their parents' need and therefore did not feel burdened with gratitude. A number said they had often thought of adopting so they could make another child as happy as they had been. A young man in a professional family said: 'Adoption is a privilege. Someone chose you, really wanted you.' The word 'lucky' was used frequently by satisfied adoptees. A former foster child with a very simple, warm-hearted family where there had been much illness over the years and almost no attention at all to housekeeping, said: 'I have been lucky. My parents showed me they loved me. My mum had the biggest heart in the world.' A successful young professional man felt lucky, said he had a reasonably happy life and still felt completely part of the family. He viewed the emotional problems of his adolescence as related not to his adoption, but to his mother's death and father's remarriage, and he said he had experienced no trauma when told of his adoptive status.

An adoptee with limited potential said: 'I was lucky and have nothing to grumble about.' He had felt close to his father when his mother had a long terminal illness and had felt very much a part of the wider family group when his father died three years before this interview. Another young man attributed his acceptance of his family relationships to the fact that his parents were completely open about the adoption, never stressed his position or made him feel different. Mary said her family had always been closer than many and she was told early 'a fairy story which later became a reality'. Several said their parents had been warm, loving and supportive and they could not fault them on anything. Jack said: 'There are no arguments I can put forward against the scheme; it was a good system and it worked well for my brother and me.'

A young man now married and the father of two children said he had always felt completely part of the family. He felt important and no different from others in the family as he was brought up the same. He thought this was why he was unconcerned about his first parents. This had been such an outstandingly happy and satisfactory adoption for all concerned, and the warm relationships within the family were so obvious, that the circumstances of the placement are worth mentioning, since they involved risks which are not usually taken in good adoption practice today. These adoptive parents had lost a set of twins (a boy and girl) at birth. They then had another daughter only a few days older than this adopted son, and they raised the two children as twins to replace those lost at birth. The children grew up happily as twins but without subterfuge, the fact of this son's adoption being known to all, as he was of nearly school-age before the adoption was legalised. This is a very closely-knit, cheerful, happy family with good relationships all round and very open about everything. They enjoy one another's company, allow for individual differences, enjoy life and are pleased to have children around. Perhaps it could be said that when a family is as warm, open and loving as this one the usual risks scarcely exist.

Just as some parents were able to feel real satisfaction in bringing up a child with certain problems or limitations, so the children were often able to feel contented with an adoptive experience that was less than perfect. There was a girl who rated her experience as satisfactory, but she was so different from her family that she said it had been impossible for her parents to understand and help her as much as they would have wished. More than one of the young men also felt they were too different for the adoptive parents to be able to understand them. Some people, while feeling overall contentment with their experience, mentioned the loneliness of their childhood and how much they had longed for brothers or sisters.

Boys more than girls had found growing up difficult or had been concerned about their identity. Some of these boys had found the overall experience satisfactory, others had not. One young man, although he considered his overall experience satisfactory, had mixed feelings about adoption, saying that 90 per cent of the time he felt fine and 'chosen', but 10 per cent of the time he felt 'cast off' by his first mother. Luckily, he had always been able to take this problem to his adoptive mother who understood and comforted him. Another whose overall experience nevertheless was very satisfactory said: 'I've always felt immense pride in being adopted. It is the illegitimacy that worries me – I have no past.'

Among those who were somewhat unhappy in their adoption was a man who had a devoted family but had taken the knowledge of his adoption hard and had let it colour the whole experience. He said: 'It's like living without an arm.' Another placed as a young baby but not legally adopted until nearly 12 years old, spoke of how he had felt more a part of the family after the court hearing, but not entirely so because he had been insecure for so long.

FACTORS ASSOCIATED WITH ADOPTEE SATISFACTION

Sex of child, age at placement, place in family
Three factors which might be expected to have some association with an adopted person's view of the experience proved to be of no significance. These were the sex of the child, his place in the adoptive family and his age at placement.

A question which often exercises adoption case committees is a child's place in the family. Should all adopters be encouraged to take two children? Will the second child be compared unfavourably with a much-loved older child? What about applicants who already have several children? Obviously, family place may be crucial for a particular child, but overall it had not been an important factor in the group under study. The adoptees who were seen were almost evenly divided into thirds – one-third who were the only child in their family, one-third who were the eldest of two or more children and one-third who were at least the second child in the family. Although several adoptees had longed for brothers and sisters, in fact, the proportion of 'only' children who were satisfied was the same as for those with siblings. In Chapter 5 it was seen that six adoptees were the fourth, fifth, or sixth child in their family and that parental satisfaction was adequate in all of these six cases. Unfortunately, only three of these adoptees could be interviewed, but these three were well satisfied with their adoption.

The age of the child at placement showed no apparent relation to adoptee satisfaction any more than it had to parental satisfaction, but as the group of adoptees we were able to see included only eight who had been placed after their first birthday we were dealing mostly with a group of children who were close in age when they were placed.

Age and social class of adoptive parents

The age of the parents, especially the mother, was important to the adoptees, and the proportion who assessed their experience as satisfactory dropped with the mother's increasing age. Nine in ten with a mother under 30 at the time of placement were satisfied with the adoption, but this was true of only two in every three whose mothers were 40 or above. An informant with parents of 40 and 45 when she was placed with them spoke like an older woman herself. She had a long-standing co-habitation which was very important to her and it had been a source of grief to her that her elderly mother was so critical of it. Another girl with parents who were 40 when they took her said she had at last matured enough to be able to accept her elderly parents and make allowances for them, but earlier she had been through a very turbulent adolescence. One of the men said his father was 'always too old for cricket and out of touch with modern trends'.

Other research findings have varied with regard to the relation between age of adoptive parents and outcome of the adoption. Some investigators have found no relation, but in one recent survey carried out in France in 1976 adult adoptees were said to 'demand' young parents for adopted children. This may have been because those adoptees had grown up with older parents, as a requirement of French law until recently made it impossible for a couple to adopt until they were so old that they were unlikely to have a child born to them. This was true in some other European countries as well, where legislation was based on Roman law which viewed adoption largely in terms of inheritance.

Table 6.2   *Adoptees' satisfaction with their experience of growing up adopted, related to social class of adoptive father*

	Social class of adoptive father										
	Social class I		*Social class II*		*Social class III*		*Social class IV*		*Social class V*		*Total*
	no.	*%*	*no.*	*%*	*no.*	*%*	*no.*	*%*	*no.*	*%*	*no.* *%*
Adoptees' experience											
Satisfactory	14	*93*	21	*72*	43	*84*	5	*56*	—	—	83 *80*
Unsatisfactory	1	*7*	8	*28*	8	*16*	4	*44*	—	—	21 *20*
Total	15	*100*	29	*100*	51	*100*	9	*100*	—	—	104* *100*

* Figures exclude one who could not be questioned on the subject.

As shown in Table 6.2 the adoptees with fathers in professional or managerial positions were those most often satisfied and the small number with fathers in semi-skilled manual work least often satisfied.

Basis of placement and time to legal adoption

The basis on which the adoptees had first been received into these homes showed no apparent relationship with their feeling of satisfaction in the experience of growing up there. However, as shown in Table 6.3, it may be noteworthy that when members of the little group placed only for fostering had found the experience satisfactory they tended somewhat more often than the others to have found it very much so. In this respect they differed from their adoptive parents. It will be recalled from Chapter 5 that the satisfied parents of these former foster children were more often only moderately satisfied. The number of 'true' foster children is of course too small to mean very much, but in the absence of a larger number this difference may be of interest.

The question as to whether original placement as a foster child with a long delay in legalisation would be associated with a less satisfying experience for the adopted person was answered in the negative. The proportion of satisfied people among those who were adopted after two years or more in their foster family was almost as great as in the group adopted more quickly. (Table 6.4). However, it should be noted that among those who were dissatisfied there were several who recalled vividly the unhappiness associated with several years of uncertainty about belonging and about their surname being different from their family's.

Table 6.3 *Adoptees' satisfaction with their experience of growing up adopted, related to basis on which they were received into their families*

	Basis on which child was received							
	Adoption only		Fostering with a view to adoption		Fostering only		Total	
	no.	%	no.	%	no.	%	no.	%
Adoptees' experience								
Very satisfactory	27	56 ⎫	25	57 ⎫	8	67 ⎫	60	58
Reasonably		⎬ 81		⎬ 80		⎬ 75		
satisfactory	12	25 ⎭	10	23 ⎭	1	8 ⎭	23	22
Mainly unsatisfactory	7	15	8	18	3	25	18	17
Very unsatisfactory	2	4	1	2	—	—	3	3
Total	48	100	44	100	12	100	104*	100

* Figures exclude one who could not be questioned on the subject.

Table 6.4 *Adoptees' satisfaction with their experience of growing up adopted, related to length of time to adoption order*

	Time to adoption order									
	Less than 1 year		1–2 years		2–5 years		5 or more years		Total	
	no.	%	no.	%	no.	%	no.	%	no.	%
Adoptees' experience										
Satisfactory	43	83	21	81	12	75	7	70	83	80
Unsatisfactory	9	17	5	19	4	25	3	30	21	20
Total	52	100	26	100	16	100	10	100	104*	100

* Figures exclude one who could not be questioned on the subject.

Community

Most of the adoptees lived in surban areas or in towns, but those who lived in villages or rural areas sometimes had felt conspicuous and 'different', especially those who had lived with the family for several years as foster children. Parents, too, in small communities had often felt their parenting ability was being scrutinised and that they were under social pressure to make the children conform. Not surprisingly, there was some relationship between the attitude of the community and adoptee satisfaction.

Relationships

As one would expect, satisfaction in the whole experience was closely associated with relationships within the adoptive family during the growing-up years. Where adoptees thought relationships within their families had been well balanced, they were more often satisfied than in families where they had felt like foster children or step-children, or even where the family life had revolved around them and made them feel too special and different. Presumably the latter focused too much attention and expectation and this responsibility weighed heavily upon them. Being treated as though born into the family was very important indeed to them and more than 90 per cent who felt this way were satisfied with their experience. In an unusual case, a young man was satisfied with his adoption, as he had always been well loved by his parents even though the extended family had allocated him an inferior status and refused to recognise him as one of them, because they feared he might one day take over the small family business.

The emotional climate in the home during the growing-up years had been important, as it is for all children, and it influenced very much the adoptees' feelings about their whole experience. If they had a family where relationships were warm and harmonious and the climate one of well-being and security throughout their childhood, nine in ten adoptees felt well satisfied with their adoption. But when the atmosphere had deteriorated later or the prevailing climate over the years had been characterised by conflict, worry or insecurity, only seven in ten now felt well satisfied.

Like most young people the adopted persons were much more often satisfied when parents had given them some freedom to follow and develop their own interests, choose their own friends and career and take some risks. This was true of George, who was very musical and appreciated very much his parents' allowing him to prepare for and pursue a career in music when it was far from their own more everyday interests; but an unforgettable example of one who was not satisfied was the man who had wanted to study art, but was required by his practical, hard-working parents to become a plumber.

Feeling close to both parents over the years was, quite naturally, clearly associated with satisfaction. All except one of the fifty-four who had felt close to both parents while growing up were satisfied with their overall experience as adopted children. Feeling close to neither parent or closer to someone else, for example, a grandparent or sibling, was likely to be associated with lack of satisfaction. But rather surprisingly five of the fifteen, who said they had not felt close to anyone while growing up, nevertheless were satisfied. We are left to suppose that they had not expected much for themselves or were simply unaware of the possibilities for close and meaningful relationships within families.

Likeness to adopters

The young adults in this study and also (as we have seen) their adoptive parents were much more often satisfied when they were able to perceive or even imagine likenesses between them. These were not necessarily thought of as similarities which under other circumstances might have been inherited from these parents, but likenesses nevertheless. They enjoyed feeling they were birds of a feather and when they did so they were virtually always satisfied with their adoption. A very large proportion were satisfied even when feeling just somewhat alike, but this could be said of only half when they were uncertain or saw in themselves no likeness to these parents (Table 6.5).

Table 6.5 *Adoptees' satisfaction with their experience of growing up adopted, related to their perception of likeness to their adoptive family*

	Feeling of likeness to adoptive family									
	Very much like		Somewhat like		Unlike or uncertain		Not covered		Total	
	no.	%	no.	%	no.	%	no.	%	no.	%
Adoptees' experience										
Satisfactory	37	97	29	85	15	52	2	67	83	80
Unsatisfactory	1	3	5	15	14	48	1	33	21	20
Total	38	100	34	100	29	100	3	100	104*	100

* Figures exclude one who could not be questioned on one of these subjects.

Communication about adoption

The question of how adopted people learn about their adoption and come to accept it is so important that it needs a chapter to itself and will be discussed fully in Chapter 9. For the moment it must suffice to give a few facts about how satisfaction was related to contentment with the information adoptees had received and to the attitudes to birth parents.

Satisfaction was found to be closely related to contentment with the information given about background. In fact 75 per cent of the people who were satisfied with their adoption were also contented with the information they had received, whereas of those who were generally dissatisfied only 14 per cent were content with what they had been told. The actual amount of information given is not the issue here. Some were content with very little while others wanted much more. No apparent relationship was found between satisfaction and how *often* the adoption was discussed within the family – this seemed to be a highly individual matter – but there *was* a clear relationship with the degree of ease and comfort people felt in being able to ask their adoptive parents for further information if they wanted it (Table 6.6).

Table 6.6　*Adoptees' satisfaction with their experience of growing up adopted, related to ease of discussion with parents*

	Adoptees' ease of discussion							
	Comfortable		Uncomfortable		Not covered		Total	
	no.	%	no.	%	no.	%	no.	%
Adoptees' experience								
Satisfactory	45	96	36	65	1	100	82	80
Unsatisfactory	2	4	19	35	–	–	21	20
Total	47	100	55	100	1	100	103*	100

* Figures exclude two who could not be questioned on the subject.

There also seemed to be a firm link between satisfied adoptees and their view of their adoptive parents' attitude towards their family of origin. Virtually all those who thought their adoptive parents had accepted their background were satisfied with their adoption, while this was true of only two-thirds when they thought the adopters had mixed feelings or were critical or disapproving of the birth parents. There had been little discussion of background in many of these families, which may be the reason nearly half did not know how their adoptive parents felt about the other parents (Table 6.7).

As we have seen, even otherwise secure and well-satisfied adoptive parents were found to have a deep-seated fear that an interest in, let alone a contact with, the birth parents would result in their losing their child's affection. The interview with the adoptees showed how unnecessary these fears really were.

The Children Act, 1975, has made the whole question of contact between adopted people and their birth parents of even greater interest than it was at the time the study took place. As Table 6.8 shows, of the 23 adoptees who expressed interest in contacting their birth parents nearly 40 per cent were dissatisfied with their adoption, whereas of the much larger number who expressed no such interest only 11 per cent were dissatisfied.

Table 6.7 *Adoptees' satisfaction with their experience of growing up adopted, related to adoptive parents' attitude to birth parents*

	Adoptive parents' attitude to birth parents									
	Accepting		Critical or mixed		Attitude unknown		Not covered		Total	
	no.	%	no.	%	no.	%	no.	%	no.	%
Adoptees' experience										
Satisfactory	30	94	11	65	38	76	4	80	83	80
Unsatisfactory	2	6	6	35	12	24	1	20	21	20
Total	32	100	17	100	50	100	5	100	104*	100

* Figures exclude one who could not be questioned on the subject.

Table 6.8 *Adoptees' satisfaction with their experience of growing up adopted, related to their current interest in contacting their birth parents*

	Interest in contact							
	No wish for contact		Unclear or rejecting		Wish for contact		Total	
	no.	%	no.	%	no.	%	no.	%
Adoptees' satisfaction								
Satisfactory	66	89	3	43	14	61	83	80
Unsatisfactory	8	11	4	57	9	39	21	20
Total	74	100	7	100	23	100	104*	100

* Figures exclude one who could not be questioned on the subject.

Problems in growing up
Adoptees described by their parents as having behaviour or personality problems while growing up were, like their parents, less often satisfied with the adoption experience than those with no such problems. This was especially pronounced among the adoptees whose behaviour had brought them to the attention of the police at one time or another. Does this suggest that delinquency or other problematic behaviour indicated dissatisfaction with the way their adoption was going?

Personal achievement
The young people we interviewed were more than twice as often found to be satisfied when they were making a good work adjustment as when they were finding little pleasure in their work and changing jobs often. Also, sons and daughters who were thought by parents to have made good use of the opportunities offered them were more often satisfied with their adoption than those who were said to have thrown them away. While nearly nine of every ten of the adoptees now employed in work classified by the Registrar General as social classes I, II or III occupations or who were in the armed forces were satisfied overall with their adoption, less than half of those in the semi-skilled and unskilled occupations classified as social classes IV or V were satisfied.

Adults who are doing well in life can probably be expected to feel positively about the growing-up experiences which helped them towards these achievements. Certainly it seems so in this study. The cause and effect relationship could not be disentangled, but there seems no doubt that a relationship does exist between the adoptees' own achievement and their overall satisfaction with their adoption. A good many parents said their most serious conflict with the child had come because of his cavalier attitude to school. Yet it seemed that parents' efforts to encourage their children to achieve qualifications or skills sometimes bore fruit and were appreciated later when sons and daughters found themselves qualified to enjoy rewarding work.

Current attitudes
Achievement and adjustment are bound to be closely related to an individual's feelings about himself. It is possible to be insecure, unhappy and self-critical while doing well. But it is much more likely that success in education, career and personal relationships will lead to a sense of personal worth and that this in turn will lead to a kind and generous attitude towards other people. In learning to value himself, in acquiring a good self-image, an adopted person has some additional tasks to complete. He has to find his identity by fusing his dual heritage and come to terms with his minority status. While he may feel secure in having been 'chosen', the reality is that his birth parents were unable or unwilling to keep him. Thus it may be seen as

inevitable that the adoptees' current concept of themselves and how much they respect the values, rights and needs of other people would be related to their satisfaction with their adoption.

More than 90 per cent of those who were thought to have a good self-image were satisfied with their adoption, and so were more than three-quarters of those who were thought to be somewhat less certain of their worth, but very few were satisfied with being adopted when they believed they were of little value or felt isolated, rejected or depressed. Almost nine in every ten who were thought by their parents to have respect for others also were contented with their adoption, compared with two in three of those whose interest in others was largely limited to what they could get from them, and compared with only one in three of those who had no respect for the rights and needs of other people.

As with the parents, most but not all of the adoptees were satisfied with their experience as adopted people. Although most of them tended not to blame this experience for whatever difficulties they were facing now or the problems they had had as children, we have seen their satisfaction linked with many factors in their life in the adoptive family. We also have seen it related to their own achievement, to the kind of adult life they are able to make for themselves and to the way they now value themselves and others.

Chapter 7

———◆———

THE ADOPTED PEOPLE'S PRESENT LIFE-ADJUSTMENT

ASSESSING ADOPTEE ADJUSTMENT

Defining the word 'adjustment' as conformance or adaptation to one's environment, in this instance to life as a young adult in Britain in the 1970s, the project staff did not feel capable of measuring this adjustment in a scientific way. The adoptees were interviewed only once by an experienced social worker in the role of research interviewer, not by a psychologist or psychiatrist, and no projective tests were given. We thought the idea of such tests might not be acceptable to some parents and therefore might reduce the number of adoptees we would be able to see. Yet in spite of these lacks, when some criteria had been established, we did feel that a carefully considered estimate could be made of the overall current adjustment, as it was described by the adoptees themselves and as it appeared to the social workers who saw them and to the project director who heard the interviews on tape. The assessment was limited to the 105 adoptees who actually took part in the research; no attempt was made to rate those whose parents alone were seen.

Criteria were formulated, each with five alternative measurements which were coded from the interview tapes, then added up, the lower the score the higher the rating. As some of the criteria were obviously more important than others, some weighting would have been desirable, but the issues became too complex and controversial to fall within the scope of this project. Nor was it possible to disentangle the interrelationships between various factors though some of these were evident. The areas covered in the assessments were: the adoptee's satisfaction with his life at the present time; self-concept; present relationship with adoptive parents; relationships with friends; views about marriage and children; use of opportunities for self-development; the adoptee's overall view of life. Coding some of these criteria required professional judgements and these were made jointly by the project director and the interviewer concerned. Each adoptee was assigned to one of four adjustment groups on the basis of the established criteria; A—excellent, B—good, C—barely adequate or marginal, D—poor. No allowance was made for differences in family background or the advantages or disadvantages some children might have started with or encountered over the years. The concern here was solely with the sort of adjustment to life the adoptees were making at the time we saw them as young adults in their twenties. However, in the case of the man who suffered from very severe epilepsy and was permanently hospitalised, the rating of 'barely adequate' was made in relation to his adjustment to the hospital environment in which he lives. It might be argued that his adjustment should be rated as 'poor' on the basis of his inability to manage outside a hospital, but on balance it was felt that he should be rated in accordance with the possibilities open to him with his handicap.

CURRENT ADJUSTMENT

Seventy-three adoptees were found to be making a good or excellent life-adjustment at this time. These 70 per cent were all making their way in the world of adults in a very creditable manner, and among them 32 people (Group A) were thought to be making an excellent adjustment. There was a young professional man with a painting done in his spare time and exhibited at the Royal Academy, and there were solicitors, doctors, scientists, social workers, nurses, teachers, secretaries, and some less well endowed who, nevertheless, were self-supporting, likeable young adults, most of them still enjoying a close and significant relationship with their adoptive family. Among those who were best adjusted nearly all had made their adoptive parents' way of life their own. Even now there was a very real *rapport* between them and their parents, though there were three exceptions to this, families where adoptees had enjoyed far more education than the adopters and had developed cultural and intellectual interests which the parents were not able to share (Table 7.1).

Table 7.1   *Adoptees' current overall adjustment as rated in the project*

Current adjustment	No.		%	
Excellent (Group A)	32 ⎱	73	31 ⎱	70
Good (Group B)	41 ⎰		39 ⎰	
Marginal (Group C)	26 ⎱	32	25 ⎱	30
Poor (Group D)	6 ⎰		5 ⎰	
Total	105		100	

In contrast to the 70 per cent who were considered to be well adjusted, there were 6 adoptees with very serious emotional and social problems who were very definitely poorly adjusted (Group D) and 26 who were classified as making a barely adequate or marginal adjustment at this time (Group C), i.e. a total of 30 per cent who were either poorly adjusted or very much at risk of becoming so. The 6 poorly adjusted were so clearly unhappy and depressed that it was noticeable in their voice, posture and facial expression, and they presented a marked contrast to the 73 mature, cheerful, self-confident young adults in Groups A and B, who gave every evidence of being well adjusted and enjoying life.

One of the six Group D cases was interviewed in prison where he was serving a three-year sentence and was very unhappy and depressed. He had been involved in delinquency since the age of 8. The adoptive mother had died before he went to school, his uninterested father somewhat later, and he was brought up by an adoptive relative who felt it was her Christian duty, but who had no enthusiasm for the task. Another young man had been looked after by his rather elderly foster mother and her relatives after the foster father died when the boy was little more than a toddler. He continued with the family on a fostering basis until a crisis precipitated his legal adoption when he was nearly adolescent. When he began to have brushes with the law, the family were embarrassed by his behaviour and when it continued they finally washed their hands of him. He no longer has a home there, drifts from one unskilled job to another and is frequently in trouble.

Also very maladjusted, but in quite a different situation, was a young man who at 24 was so tied to his extremely domineering and possessive mother that he seemed to have no identity apart from her and was like a puppet on a string. Two others were back home after ill-advised and hasty marriages had broken down. Both had serious emotional problems. One was drinking heavily, was promiscuous and seemed largely out of touch with reality. The other was extremely withdrawn and uncommunicative, and totally irresponsible towards the family he had established. Both men were very immature, unhappy and preoccupied with the subject of their adoption, which they had learned of quite late and never fully understood or accepted.

The only young woman whose adjustment was definitely poor was a girl of limited intelligence who was supporting herself by unskilled work but continuing to live at home with her ageing and dissatisfied adoptive parents and her illegitimate son. She had been jilted by the baby's father and was now rejected by her parents. She was sullen and depressed and left to her parents the care and responsibility for her child.

The 26 adoptees whose adjustment was rated as 'barely adequate' were just that – they were coping much better than the unfortunate 6 just described, but their adjustment was precarious and it seemed that it would not take much misfortune or frustration to upset it. For example, there was a young man who had been at odds with his parents for years, a lone drifter, who had recently joined a religious sect where he found like-minded friends and a job. At the time we saw him he was doing better than he had ever done before, but he is inclined to test people to the limit and then find them wanting, and we wondered if this latest commitment would endure. Then there was the highly competitive young man who tended to ridicule people who were committed to anything or anyone and was suspicious of the motives of others. There was a handicapped young woman who was impatient and could not get on with people but felt useful and contented as housekeeper for her aged father. Her father, quite naturally, wondered what would happen to her after his death. Several adoptees in this 'marginal' group were very dependent upon their marriage or current cohabitation for what security they now felt in their lives. There were also two or three men who were quite well adjusted to their authoritarian role in the armed forces or the police but were suspicious and intolerant, and it seemed unlikely their adjustment would survive without the props provided by the firm structure within which they were working. Although the adjustment of any of the adoptees might have been somewhat different if they had been interviewed at a different time, say six months or a year earlier or later, this was especially so in regard to those in adjustment Group C, where some change in circumstances might have improved their adjustment or caused it to deteriorate further.

It is a major problem of adoption follow-up research that there are no adequate yardsticks against which to judge the performance of adoptive families. No one knows what proportion of parents are satisfied with the children born to them, or vice versa. No one can say what proportion of young adults would be considered well-adjusted by the rather stringent criteria which we used in this project. A comparison group of non-adopted people would, of course, provide some answers. Some other studies have compared younger adopted children with their schoolmates and in due course the longitudinal study now in progress at the National Children's Bureau in London will provide some valuable data, but the cost and technical problems in finding a properly matched sample of adopted adults have defeated all researchers so far.

There has been a tendency among social workers, and to a lesser extent in the general population, to expect a successful adoption to be perfect and to equate problems with failure. As we have already seen, adoptive parents and children could cope with a wide range of difficulties while feeling generally satisfied with each other. Nevertheless, it certainly is to be expected that some children will turn out better than others and they will not all become equally well-adjusted adults. It is interesting, though, that the proportion of well-adjusted adoptees in this study was so nearly the same as in the very first follow-up of grown-up adopted and foster children more than 50 years ago (Theis, 1924).

Relation between adjustment and satisfaction
In most cases adjustment and satisfaction went hand in hand, as might be expected, but there were some exceptions. Three adopted people who were well-adjusted (Group B) were not really satisfied with their adoption. One of these had suffered from a good deal of friction within the adoptive family and had been required to leave school early in order to help out in a relative's

shop; another had found life so restricted in the home of a very religious family that she had found it necessary to rebel in order to survive; the third, a rather intellectual man, felt he had little in common with his doting parents.

There were also five adoptees who were well adjusted (one in Group A, four in Group B) even though their parents were not satisfied with them, or perhaps this should be said the other way round – that five families were dissatisfied even though their children were now well adjusted. In each of these cases parental expectations had been unrealistic and attempts at moulding the child to a predetermined pattern had failed. The children had been able to achieve a good adjustment but not one that was satisfactory to their parents. On the other hand, the parents of well over half of the adoptees who were now poorly or marginally adjusted had, nevertheless, found the adoption a rewarding experience, so it seems that for some parents, at least, their child's problems of adult personal and social maladjustment were not sufficient to make them feel overall dissatisfaction with the adoption. In a few cases it was felt that parents refused to recognise the seriousness of the problem, perhaps because they were too limited in their understanding to be able to do so. In some other cases the adoptee's problems quite obviously confirmed the parents' prejudices or fitted into their personality needs in such a way as to be gratifying to the parents, for example, an overprotective and possessive mother and her very dependent son, or a father who acts out his own unacceptable drives by subtly encouraging his son's anti-social behaviour.

In seven cases involving four boys and three girls the outcome of the adoption was negative in all three measures of outcome – in terms of an adoptee's current adjustment, his dissatisfaction with his experience as an adopted child of this family and his adoptive parents' dissatisfaction with their experience.

FACTORS RELATED TO CURRENT ADJUSTMENT

Sex of adoptees, age at placement, background factors
The current adjustment of nearly two-thirds of the men and three-quarters of the women was classified as A (excellent) or B (good). The difference really came in A with only one in four of the men but two in five of the women coming into this group. It is perhaps noteworthy that five of the six adoptees making the poorest adjustment and classified as D were men. (Two of these were among the eight men whose parents had been very dissatisfied.)

In other adoption studies, too, somewhat more women than men were found to be making a good adjustment. Jaffee and Fanshel (1973, p. 71) found this to be so and theorised that the sex of a child might have a different meaning for some parents in the context of adoption than it would in biological parenthood, in that adopted sons might not be viewed as rightful heirs and that in some families, therefore, boys would be exposed to ambivalent attitudes and possibly to disguised rejection. In studies of younger adoptees several other investigators have found boys making a more problematical adjustment than girls, especially in the area of school attitudes and achievement (Witmer *et al.*, 1963; Bohman, 1970; Seglow *et al.*, 1972), although Kornitzer (1968, p. 164) found in her group of adoptees, who were of widely varying ages, that 'the girls had a far larger proportion of bad or failed adoptions than the boys'.

Just as in the other two measures of outcome – the satisfaction of parents and adoptees – there was no consistent pattern in this part of the study to support the idea that age at placement was linked with later adult adjustment, although this is at variance with some other studies especially those based on child guidance clinic cases. (Once again it must be remembered that the current study dealt almost entirely with children placed before they were 1 year old, so the difference was usually one of months rather than years.) Nor was any apparent relationship found between present adoptee adjustment and earlier experience of life in a residential nursery, or with the total number of living arrangements, or the number of foster home placements before this one. The six adoptees who were now making the poorest adjustment, as well as nearly three-quarters of the marginally adjusted, had never been in any other foster family, so their poor adjustment could not be related to loss of other foster parents. Some other studies with more background data available particularly Lawder (1969, p. 104) found that such background factors as age at adoption placement, pre-adoption placement history, psychological evaluation and rating of emotional deprivation showed very little relationship to later functioning. In 1970 Kadushin demonstrated the reversibility of early trauma in a group of children adopted when over 5 years of age, and in 1977 Tizard showed the capacity adopted children have for overcoming the effects of residential care. In these studies it seemed that adoption had provided an experience which these children had hitherto lacked.

Basis of placement and time to legal adoption
The data provided no clear answer to the query as to whether children received into the family first as foster children (usually with a view to adoption) are likely to become as well-adjusted adults as those placed with their families directly for adoption. No apparent relationship was seen between method of placement and overall adult adjustment. However, among the adoptees who were now doing well there was a tendency for those who had first been received by the family on a fostering basis to be making only a moderately good rather than an excellent adjustment, while among those not doing so well those first fostered were more often the ones who were making a really poor adjustment. Looking at the worst-adjusted group (Group D), five of the six are found to have been received by these families first on a fostering basis (Table 7.2). It was noticed that the former foster

children less often seemed to be using their full potential, were less often fully stretched, perhaps because some of their families had expected less of them and had provided only a limited amount of encouragement and stimulation to develop special abilities and gifts. Conversely, it is likely that some others were now making at least a reasonably good adjustment just because not too much had been expected of them and the relationships within the home had been so comfortable and accepting.

Table 7.2 *Adoptees' current adjustment, related to basis on which they were received into their families*

	Basis on which child was received					
	Adoption only		Fostering only or with a view to adoption		Total	
	no.	%	no.	%	no.	%
Current adjustment						
Excellent (A)	18	37 } 71	14	25 } 68	32	31
Good (B)	17	35 }	24	43 }	41	39
Marginal (C)	13	26 } 29	13	23 } 32	26	25
Poor (D)	1	2 }	5	9 }	6	5
Total	49	100	56	100	105	100

The project staff had wondered if the mere fact of living a long time in the family before legal adoption might be associated with poor adult adjustment because of the protracted anxiety suffered by parents and children over the uncertainty of their situation. Plenty of this anxiety was seen but the figures, nevertheless, do not show any significant relationship between adult adjustment and late legalisation of the adoption (Table 7.3).

Contact between adopters and birth mother
There has been much speculation among social workers about the effect of adoptive parents meeting the birth mother. Among the 105 adoptees who were interviewed there were 34 whose adoptive parents had met the mother, usually when she visited in the home while they were fostering the child prior to legal adoption. No apparent relationship was found between these meetings and the adoptees' adult adjustment. In a few other cases there had been direct correspondence (not through the agency) between the adopters and the mother or grandmother, but no face to face meeting, with the result that these adopters' whole perception of the birth mother had been derived

from one or two letters or greeting cards from which they ever after thought of her as 'immature', 'illiterate', 'emotional' or 'a lovely girl'.

What did seem to be associated with adjustment was the *reaction* of the adoptive parents over the years to meeting or not meeting the birth mother. Those who were glad it had happened as it did much more often had children who were well adjusted as young adults. Of course the adopters' feeling about this may have altered over the years, and their feeling at the time they were interviewed may have been coloured by the very fact of the kind of adjustment an adoptee was making or by their own satisfaction with the whole experience. Quite naturally, if things had turned out well one might be glad they happened as they did, whereas an unhappy outcome would make one feel that if events had been different the result might have been better. Whatever the reason, this seems a good example of feelings mattering more than facts in adoption outcome.

Table 7.3   *Adoptees' current adjustment, related to time in family before adoption order*

	Length of time to legal adoption									
	Less than 1 year		1–2 years		2–5 years		5 or more years		Total	
	no.	%	no.	%	no.	%	no.	%	no.	%
Current adjustment										
Excellent (A)	19	36	7	27	3	19	3	30	32	31
Good (B)	20	38	10	38	7	44	4	40	41	39
Marginal (C)	13	24	7	27	4	25	2	20	26	25
Poor (D)	1	2	2	8	2	12	1	10	6	5
Total	53	100	26	100	16	100	10	100	105	100

The adoptive family setting
Age of adoptive parents. Quite a few people mentioned the age gap between themselves and their adoptive parents. Some felt it was a handicap, particularly at adolescence, to have older parents. Others were finding it hard as young adults, because they were just getting started in a career or with a family of their own at the time when their parents were already suffering the infirmities of old age and needed to be able to depend on them for assistance of one kind or another. Many adoptees mentioned their feeling of responsibility towards their parents' well-being. But though (as explained in the previous chapter) the figures show a definite link between

adoptee satisfaction and the age of their parents, they show only a very marginal association between parental age and the young adults' present adjustment. Mothers who were in their twenties and fathers who were in their thirties at the time the child in the study was placed with them now had the largest proportion of well-adjusted adoptees while both fathers and mothers who were 40 or more had the smallest, but the difference was not great enough to be significant. Two adoptive mothers were over 50 when they first fostered the child they later adopted and, not too surprisingly, neither of these adoptees was now making a good adjustment.

Family place. No relationship was shown between adjustment and family place. Indeed, the presence or absence of siblings, whether older or younger, natural born or adopted, did not seem to be important to later adoptee adjustment. As might be expected, where there were older children in the family the adoptee was much more often found to be well adjusted if he felt these brothers and sisters had loved and accepted him than if they had been indifferent or jealous, but adjustment did not seem to be much related to the attitude of younger siblings.

Social class. A factor which did seem to be closely related to adult adjustment was the occupation of the adoptive father with its associated social class connotation and life-style. When fathers were employed in occupations classified as social class I, the adoptees were now more likely to be making a good or excellent adjustment than when fathers were in any other occupational group. Table 7.4 shows that all but one of the fifteen

Table 7.4 *Adoptees' current adjustment, related to social class of the adoptive fathers*

	Social class of adoptive father											
	Social class I		Social class II		Social class III		Social class IV		Social class V		Total	
	no.	%	no.	%	no.	%	no.	%	no.	%	no.	%
Current adjustment												
Excellent (A)	6	40 ⎫93	8	27 ⎫60	16	31 ⎫70	2	22 ⎫56	—	—	32	31 ⎫70
Good (B)	8	53 ⎭	10	33 ⎭	20	39 ⎭	3	34 ⎭	—	—	41	39 ⎭
Marginal (C)	1	7	11	37	12	24	2	22	—	—	26	25
Poor (D)	—	—	1	3	3	6	2	22	—	—	6	5
Total	15	*100*	30	*100*	51	*100*	9	*100*	—	—	105	*100*

adoptees with fathers in social class I occupations were in adjustment groups A or B in contrast to only 60 per cent of class II, 70 per cent of class III and 56 per cent of class IV (five of these nine adoptees). In earlier chapters it was noted that the adoptive father's occupation seemed to be a factor in the satisfaction of the children but not the parents; here we see it related to the adoptees' adjustment in adult life. This finding readily lends itself to the criticism that social workers and research workers are poorly equipped because of their middle-class bias to compare the adjustment of people in different classes, but it will be recalled that these adjustments were rated on the basis of criteria thought to be applicable to individuals in any socio-economic group.

We are not able to explain why adoptees in professional and managerial families much more often achieved a satisfactory life-adjustment than those in any other occupational group. In most cases they had more advantages than adoptees in social group IV, but they also had more pressures, and most of the advantages and pressures would apply to those in semi-professional as well as to professional and managerial families.

Kornitzer (1968, p. 170) found the outcome poorest when adopters were in social class II and she attempted to explain this by saying that these people 'tended to be more idealistic in their expectations and under greater compulsion to be seen to be succeeding in all their undertakings'. No doubt in social class I the position is more secure. In America, Jaffee and Fanshel (1970, p. 309) found that children who grew up in higher-status families (presumably comparable to social classes I and II in Britain) had tended to have more personality problems while growing up than those raised in lower-status families. However, Theis (1924, p. 110), McWhinnie (1967, p. 259) and Kadushin (1970, p. 209) found the social and economic level of the homes unrelated to outcome. This difference in findings leads us to the belief that there are much more important factors than the occupation and social class of the parents as determinants of adoptee adjustment, and that these need to be looked at in combination with various other factors (for example, the quality of parenting), which taken together may influence the long-term outcome in adoption.

Relationships and care
Assessing the kind of care they had received in the adoptive home, all but one of the thirty-two best-adjusted adoptees (Group A) felt they had received an abundance of love and affection from both parents. So did more than four in five of the others with a good adjustment (Group B). However, less than half with a barely adequate adjustment felt both parents had been warm and affectionate towards them, and only one of the six poorly adjusted thought so. This last was a young man, mentioned elsewhere, who had known a suffocating kind of affection from an overprotective mother.

The overriding importance of love as the basis for emotional health is once again demonstrated by these factors. If further evidence is needed there is the additional finding that of the 14 adopted people who felt their homes had lacked real warmth and affection (though they were given good physical care), 10 were now marginally or poorly adjusted to life.

Relationships in the family are so central to any consideration of adoption that they need a chapter to themselves. But in connection with adoptee adjustment two further crucial factors must be noted. The emotional climate in the home and the young person's estimate of his status in the family while growing up were both closely linked with present adjustment. Where there had been an atmosphere of well-being and security in the home four in five children had grown up into well-adjusted adults. Only a little more than half were now doing well if they came from homes characterised by conflict, worry, insecurity or pessimism. When they felt they had been treated as though they had been born into the family four in five were now well adjusted. Of the ten who felt they had always held an inferior position only one could now be considered a well-adjusted person (Table 7.5).

Table 7.5   *Adoptees' current adjustment, related to their own view of their status in the family*

	Adoptees' view of their status in their adoptive family									
	As natural child		As foster or step-child		Other		Not covered		Total	
	no.	%	no.	%	no.	%	no.	%	no.	%
Current adjustment										
Excellent (A) or good (B)	70	80	1	10	2	33	—	—	73	70
Marginal (C) or poor (D)	17	20	9	90	4	67	2	100	32	30
Total	87	100	10	100	6	100	2	100	105	100

Events in the family
By the time this study took place 33 of the adoptees had lost a parent through death or divorce. For seven of them, these events occurred before they were 10 years old. One would have expected to find a relationship between parental loss and the adoptee's adult adjustment but this was not so. If the study had been done earlier, while the young people were in their teens, the results might well have been different, since many of them spoke of the

trauma and distress caused by death or divorce in their family, and it was clear that they had often felt this much more deeply than the remaining parent realised.

During the years these adoptees were growing up, fewer women worked outside the home than do so today. It is also unlikely that at this time adoption agencies would have accepted working mothers as adoptive parents. Thus, among the 160 families in the project there were only 9 instances of an adoptive mother working full-time for as much as a year before the child concerned reached the age of 12. In 30 other families the mother worked part-time. In fact, there seemed to be no relationship between this and adult adoptee adjustment. A much larger proportion of the adoptees' families had experienced severe or chronic illness of either a parent or another child, but there was no general link between family ill-health and the young adults' adjustment, even though in individual instances it might have had a serious effect.

Financial hardship did not figure much in these families, partly no doubt because an adequate income would have been made a requirement for adoption by both the agencies and the courts, and partly because in the 1950s and 1960s living standards were rising and unemployment was seldom a problem. As might be expected, there were few instances of poor housekeeping (that shibboleth of early work in home-finding) and those few were not associated with poor adjustment on the part of the adoptees.

Table 7.6   *Adult adjustment of adoptees, related to their perception of likeness to their adoptive family*

	Feeling of likeness to adoptive family								
	Very much like		Somewhat like		Unlike or uncertain		Not covered		Total	
	no.	%	no.	%	no.	%	no.	%	no.	%
Current adjustment										
Excellent (A)	21	55	8	24	2	7	1	25	32	31
Good (B)	16	42	16	47	9	31	—	—	41	39
Marginal (C)	1	3	10	29	12	41	3	75	26	25
Poor (D)	—	—	—	—	6	21	—	—	6	5
Total	38	100	34	100	29	100	4	100	105	100

Similarity to adopters
Just as the satisfaction that parents as well as adoptees felt in their experience of adoption was clearly related to their own idea of how much

they were alike, so adult adjustment also was related to this perception of likeness. All but one of the adoptees who felt very much like their adoptive parents were now well adjusted, and so were nearly three-quarters of those who saw themselves as somewhat like the family, but only a little over a third were making a good adjustment when they thought they were not at all like them or were uncertain about this. It should be noted that not one of the six poorly-adjusted adoptees felt he was anything like his adoptive family (Table 7.6).

Several people mentioned with obvious pleasure how much they were like one or both of their adoptive parents. One stressed the importance of 'matching' in adoption and said rather smugly how unfortunate it would have been for him and for his adoptive parents if he had been placed with an 'ordinary' family instead of with intelligent people like himself or if his adoptive parents had been given a slow child. Some said they were like their parents in appearance in that they were tall or short, fair or brunette, walked or talked in the same way or that they were alike in temperament, talents or interests. Others less well adjusted and less satisfied with their experience pointed out how entirely different they were from the adopters. A young man felt he was very much more intelligent than his parents, although up to that time he had not used this gift to acquire any higher educational qualifications, and another quite rightly perceived himself as much more academic, introspective and artistic than the adoptive parents. One of the girls, too, had always felt very different from her family, who were very warm-hearted, outgoing people, and although she loved them dearly she had never felt able to communicate with them on a deep level and had never tried to develop the very real artistic talent she showed as a child. A very dark complexioned, short, stocky man felt very different from his tall, rather fair parents and showed anxiety about his unknown ethnic background.

Communication about adoption

An important aspect of family relationships which was associated with later adjustment concerned the disclosure of the child's adoptive status and his understanding of it. The young adults seen in this project were more often well adjusted if they had not only known but really grasped the meaning of their adoptive status before starting school or if they had gradually come to an understanding of their position through discussion with their parents. However, the way the child learned about it was more important than the timing of the revelation. When their parents had helped them to understand, more than four in five adoptees were rated as well adjusted (Groups A and B), but only two in five were so rated when the understanding had come about in any other way.

Contentment with the information given them about adoption and background was found to be linked with adjustment as it had been with overall satisfaction. More than three-quarters of the well adjusted were contented with what had been disclosed to them compared with only a quarter of the others, and it is worth noting that five of the six making the poorest adjustment were dissatisfied with what they had been told.

The difficulty adoptive families have over discussing this essential topic is highlighted by the fact that, even among the best adjusted young adults, one in four was still not comfortable about raising with their parents the subject of background or the circumstances surrounding the adoption. Nevertheless, comfort in raising the subject or being able to ask questions was linked with adjustment, for in the less well-adjusted groups the proportion showing discomfort was much higher and indeed included all six of those poorly adjusted enough to be classified in Group D. In fact three of these had learned of their adoption in some other way and had *never* been able to discuss it with their parents.

Frequency of discussion did not seem linked with adjustment; it was the feelings behind the communication that mattered. When adoptive parents had been worried about something in the child's background or were afraid the agency might have withheld something from them, only a little over half the children had grown into well-adjusted adults compared with three-quarters in families who said they had never had anxieties about background.

Table 7.7 *Adoptees' current adjustment, related to their current interest in contacting birth parents*

	Interest in contact							
	No wish for contact		*Unclear or rejecting*		*Wish for contact*		*Total*	
	no.	%	no.	%	no.	%	no.	%
Current adjustment								
Excellent (A) or Good (B)	63	84	1	14	9	39	73	70
Marginal (C) or Poor (D)	12	16	6	86	14	61	32	30
Total	75	100	7	100	23	100	105	100

A feeling that parents disapproved of the adoptee's origins was associated with poor or marginal adjustment. Only half of those who thought their adopters disapproved of their birth parents were now getting along well in life.

Those adopted people who felt much interest in their birth parents – either wanting to contact them or else feeling rejecting or hostile towards them — were much more often making a poor or marginal adult adjustment than the others who had only a slight interest, or none at all, in their birth parents and entertained no desire to contact them (Table 7.7). Following on to this it was found that nearly half the less well-adjusted adoptees did not see their adopters as their real parents, or at least were unsure about it, whereas all except one of the well adjusted felt certain the adoptive parents were the real ones.

Table 7.8 *Adoptees' current adjustment, related to earlier problems of personality or behaviour*

	Earlier problems					
	Problems		No problems		Total	
	no.	%	no.	%	no.	%
Current adjustment						
Excellent (A)	10 }	55	20 }	89	30	30
Good (B)	21 }		20 }		41	40
Marginal (C)	19	34	5	11	24	24
Poor (D)	6	11	—	—	6	6
Total	56	100	45	100	101*	100

* In tables where information from interviews with adoptees is crossed with information from parent interviews only 101 adoptees are included, since the parents were not seen in the other four cases.

Problems in growing up
Poor or barely adequate adult adjustment appeared to be closely associated with earlier personality or behaviour problems. Nine in every ten of the adoptees whose parents described them as free of these problems while growing up were now well adjusted, whereas nearly half of those who had shown such problems earlier were still having difficulties. Of course, looking at it another way this means that half of those who had problems earlier have nevertheless achieved a good adjustment as adults. However, all six of the adoptees (Group D) who were now making a really poor adjustment were said to have had personality or behaviour problems when they were younger and, unfortunately, only one of them had received any professional help (Table 7.8).

Personal achievement
The ratings for adjustment were not made on the basis of educational success or prestigious employment and, as social workers, the project staff

Table 7.9 Adoptees' current adjustment, related to classification of their own employment

	Classification of adoptees' own employment													
	Social class I		Social class II		Social class III		Social class IV		Social class V		Not in classified employment (forces housewives etc.)		Total	
	no.	%	no.	%	no.	%	no.	%	no.	%	no.	%	no.	%
Current adjustment														
Excellent (A)	7	64	8	40	9	26	—	—	—	—	8	31	32	31
Good (B)	4	36	8	40	15	43	3	38	1	20	10	38	41	39
Marginal (C)	—	—	4	20	11	31	2	25	3	60	6	23	26	25
Poor (D)	—	—	—	—	—	—	3	37	1	20	2	8	6	5
Total	11	100	20	100	35	100	8	100	5	100	26	100	105	100

making the assessments tended to be biased towards concern for quality of relationships rather than material advancement. Nevertheless, the findings show a quite remarkable degree of association between the adoptees' adjustment and their level of education and occupational standing. This whole subject proved interesting enough to deserve a chapter to itself, but the main points about adjustment need to be made here.

The figures show a downward trend in good adjustment in relation to educational attainment from over 90 per cent of university students or graduates all the way to a low of 56 per cent of the adoptees with no academic or vocational qualifications. Although a surprisingly large number of these young adults said they had disliked school, many stuck it out and even went on to higher education with the result that they were now working in professional, semi-professional, or managerial occupations classified by the Registrar General as social class I or II. Those in social class I jobs were all without exception making a good or even an excellent overall adjustment to life and so was a large majority of those in social class II or III, but of those working in semi-skilled manual work considerably less than half could be rated as well adjusted, and among the five who were doing unskilled work only one was considered a well-adjusted person. Students, housewives of various levels of educational achievement and people in the armed forces tended to be getting along well. As Table 7.9 shows, no one making an excellent adjustment was in semi-skilled or unskilled manual work, while of the six adoptees who were making the poorest overall adjustment to life, four were employed in these occupations and the other two were not presently employed.

More important, though less surprising, the adoptees who were well adjusted tended to be happy in their work, but the others much less often found pleasure in it and more of them changed jobs frequently. It probably can be assumed that the adoptees' work-adjustment was contributing to their overall life-adjustment, but it also is likely that their general life-adjustment made a difference to the kind of employment they were able to get and their satisfaction with it.

Summing up, it can be said that the current adjustment of these young adults who had been adopted as children was found to be associated with their experience of relationships within their adoptive families and also with their own response to what these parents had been able to offer them. Their early life before this placement and the basis on which they were received into the families bore less relationship to their present life-adjustment than might have been expected.

PART THREE

———◆———

THE ADOPTIVE FAMILY

Chapter 8

---◆---

CONTACT BETWEEN ADOPTERS AND BIRTH PARENTS

CONTACTS BEFORE LEGAL ADOPTION

In most agency adoptions the birth mother and the new parents do not know each other, or if the agency does arrange a meeting it is brief and likely to be more of an introduction than an opportunity to get acquainted. But in this study with its large group of foster parent adopters, 43 families were interviewed in which the birth mother had visited while the child was in the home on a fostering basis. In 34 of these 43 families the adopted person was also interviewed. We were particularly interested to find out more about the effect of these visits and whether they had proved helpful in dispelling fantasies or had merely created additional anxiety. As it turned out, no really clear-cut patterns emerged, but we were given some vivid descriptions of what had gone on 20 to 25 years ago and the use and misuse to which the contacts had been put. This chapter contains examples of the wide variety of reactions which sometimes resulted from quite similar situations.

Some mothers had visited only once or twice, others several times, and in a few cases of late legalisation a mother had visited as often as once a month for several years. These visits took on different meanings in individual situations. Some adopters developed a very warm relationship with the young mother and they had her to spend a weekend or longer with them or they would take the child to visit her occasionally. The purpose seemed to be to let the mother know how well the child was getting along hoping that this would influence her to decide on adoption. It was not aimed at keeping the birth mother's image alive in the child or developing the relationship between them as might be the case in other fostering situations where the mother or relatives planned to have the child returned to them. Occasionally, the adoptive mother played a maternal role with a birth mother who felt rejected by her own parents because of her out-of-wedlock pregnancy. In one case the roles were reversed, when a somewhat older and more mature natural mother took the adoptive mother and also the small child to her home in another part of the country to recuperate from an illness. In two families the adoptive parents rather resented that the natural mother seemed to use their home as somewhere to go on her days off from work but did not show much interest in the baby.

Many adopters liked the birth mother, saw her as 'a lovely girl' or 'a girl from a good home', but one adoptive father referred to her as 'a stupid little bitch', and a few others were so intimidated by her power to withhold her consent to adoption that they scarcely saw her as an individual.

An over-anxious adoptive family with a natural mother visiting had heard of a foster child (not legally adopted) whose birth parents were said to have come and claimed him from his foster parents at the age of 15 'when he was old enough to work'. This story made such a lasting impression on them that after the legal adoption they went to live in New Zealand and only returned to England when the boy was 18. This family has suffered from lack of any real feeling of entitlement and some remnants of the anxiety persist even now. In contrast, in a family where the mother visited four times and for several months refused her consent, the adoptive mother did not feel threatened and said the visits even increased her feeling of entitlement to the child, since she could see that this young mother 'did not want the baby for keeps and was just playing about'.

A woman who had been led to believe her foster child would be available for adoption felt she could not go on caring for the little girl unless the birth mother was prepared to consent to adoption. She told the mother this on her third visit and the mother then dropped out of the picture, but at 16 the girl wrote to her mother asking for her consent to the foster parents' adopting her, and after a meeting with the girl the mother gave her consent. In another family where the mother had visited only once and had not answered the foster family's letters seeking her consent to adoption, the foster father journeyed to the family home in another part of the country to try to get her consent. At this meeting the mother's parents and siblings sided with the foster father and made it almost impossible for her to withhold her consent any longer. This was another case where the adopters certainly must have doubted their entitlement to the child, and whether because of this or not, the marriage broke down and the boy left home at 15 and never returned.

Another family had taken a foster child believing she would be available for adoption, but the mother did not give her consent for six years, and each time she visited it was clear how much she loved and wanted the child. When the legal adoption was finally completed the first mother sent a 'lovely letter', but this made the adoptive mother feel even more guilty. Quite understandably, this adoptive mother was continually aware of the little girl as someone else's child.

It was quite a different situation in the direct adoptions, where there was no question of the mother visiting since she did not know the name or address of the new parents. Nevertheless, five of these families did have (or thought they had) a fleeting contact with the child's natural mother or grandmother before the adoption was completed, and one of them thought the mother had passed them on the street three years later at a holiday resort.

In one case the adopters were introduced to the birth mother and in another to the grandmother at the agency office on the day of placement because the natural families made this a condition of handing over the babies. These adopters were unprepared for the meeting and one of them had almost completely blotted it out, remembering only that they had assured the birth mother that the baby would have good care. Two others saw the mother at the adoption court hearing and another family were convinced that they had seen the mother at the agency office, but were not introduced to her, on the day they had taken the child. They were favourably impressed with the girl and later found this a great help in interpreting her to the child.

Twenty-nine, three in five, of these forty-eight adopters who met their child's first mother were glad they had done so. Eight, fewer than one in five, were sorry and wished they had not met; the others saw it as unimportant. Of the one hundred and twelve adopters who did not meet the mother or any member of her family, only eight regretted this or thought now that it might have been better if they had. In seven other families the parents disagreed about this, the mothers saying they would like to have met the child's birth mother and the fathers saying they would have been opposed to this. Those who would like to have met the birth mother, or now in retrospect thought it was a good idea, held this view for a variety of reasons and it seems doubtful if some of them would have wanted it at the time. Where there had been difficulties with the child over the years, some people thought meeting might have helped them to understand the child better. Also, in one case where everything had turned out well the adopters thought meeting would have shown them 'what would come out in the child' and presumably would have allayed any anxiety.

Unfortunately, the opinions of the adoptees themselves could be only theoretical in most cases, as very few knew if there had been any meeting between their adoptive parents and their birth mother, even when there had been several contacts, and even fewer had any firm or thoughtful opinion on this subject. Parents sometimes said meeting had made it easier to tell the adoptee about his birth mother, yet most had never told the child about the meeting or made the most of it to satisfy his curiosity.

There were only two adopted people who, knowing their parents actually had met the birth mother, felt it would have been better if they had not done so. One of these was the young man whose parents so feared the possibility of reclaim that they felt it necessary to take him halfway round the world to make sure the birth mother would not find him. Another was the girl mentioned above, whose adoptive mother found it difficult to feel any entitlement to her because she had seen how reluctant the natural mother was to part with the child. This girl felt the meetings had made her adoptive mother anxious and over-protective.

Most adoptees did not know if there had been a meeting and many of them felt it was unimportant, but 14 would have liked their adoptive parents to have known their birth mother. Most, but not all, of these were people who had had an unsatisfactory experience of adoption and thought a meeting might have helped in some way. One unhappy young man, mentioned earlier, who felt abused by his father and rejected by his mother, thought that if his two sets of parents had met, his 'proper parents' might have kept an eye on him when things were not going well for him. Some others were mainly glad the adopters had not met the birth mother. One of these said his adoptive mother could not have coped with a meeting, and another said his adoptive father could not have coped as he was 'far too emotional'. A third thought it would have been too upsetting, and a fourth was glad the adopters had not met her first mother but had 'just accepted me as me', while a fifth said it would have been hard for her adoptive parents because she was so much their child.

CONTACTS AFTER LEGAL ADOPTION

There has often been speculation about whether birth mothers are likely to seek out or try to contact their children in any way once legal adoption has has been completed. Some adopters fear this possibility even though they know the adoption agency has not given their name or address to anyone in the biological family. But when a foster child is adopted, the birth mother is very likely to know the address of the foster parents and she may even have visited in their home and corresponded with them, as we have just seen in the foster parent adoptions in this study. Indeed, the mother of one adoptee in the study consented to the adoption on condition that she could keep in touch, and this she did until the boy was 3 years old and she herself was married and had another child. In another case the boy was 9 when the legal adoption took place and the birth mother had been visiting regularly over the years. The adoptive mother offered to send the birth mother a photograph of this boy every year and did so for two years until the adoptive father said the boy was now theirs and the time had come to forget about his other mother.

In all there were 16 cases in which letters, cards or photographs were exchanged between the adoptive parents and the birth mother in the years after the legal adoption, but these people did not meet again. Two were direct adoptions and in one of these cases the contact was through the agency. This mother wrote once and then sent a gift to the child at Christmas, but the agency advised the adopters not to reply and there was no further contact. In the second case a letter was received directly from the biological mother on the child's first birthday asking for a photograph. The adopters had never met her and were distressed to find that she had learned their address from the matron at the nursery where the adoption agency had sent them to collect the child. They became so fearful that the mother might suddenly appear on their doorstep that after sending a photograph they hurriedly moved away from the area.

Among the foster parent adopters there was often a willingness, sometimes even an expectation, that a birth mother would write once or twice soon after the legal adoption, that she would not necessarily sever the relationship with the child or with them all at once, but they usually found it trying in the few instances where it continued for several years or after the mother had married and had other children. In fact most mothers who kept in touch at all did so only briefly or until their own lives had become more settled. If they had felt close to the adopters earlier in the placement they sometimes brought a new husband to meet them or to see the child. In some of these cases the relationship had become one between the adopters and birth mother and seemed no longer to have very much to do with the child.

There was one case where a foster parent adopter received a letter from the birth mother when the child was 12 years old, and another in which a young man received a twenty-first birthday card from his birth mother. In the latter case the adopters appeared to find this more upsetting than the boy, who took it very calmly. Another family was really traumatised by receiving a letter from the birth mother just a year before the research interview when the adopted son was 23. The mother had visited in their home two or three times before the legal adoption and they were still living at the same address. They were alarmed to learn that she had just returned to the area, and was living in a nearby city. Not knowing how to reply they consulted a solicitor, who wrote for them reminding the mother that the boy was happily adopted and that in consenting to the adoption the mother had agreed not to try to contact him again. Following this letter nothing further was heard from the mother. As the son had not been an easy child and had now settled down to a fairly good adjustment, the family were particularly anxious not to take any chance of upsetting him. They welcomed the research interview as an opportunity to talk the situation over with someone outside their family and community, but they had not told the son about his first mother's letter and they were unwilling to risk an interview for him at this time.

There was one very unusual incident in a family which had only reluctantly allowed the birth mother to visit while she was deciding whether or not to relinquish the child. This mother corresponded with the adoptive mother for two years after the adoption, then nothing further was heard from her. But when the son was 13 a policeman appeared at the door saying there had been an inquiry about the 'foster child' and he must see him. When the adoptive mother said the boy was no longer a foster child, but had been legally adopted some years before this, the policeman said that in that case all would be well if she would show him the adoption order. The papers were shown and the policeman took his leave. The adoptive mother was convinced that the birth mother was checking up on the boy in this way and wanted to reclaim him. Whether this was the reason for the police inquiry is not known. Whatever the explanation, it was an unpleasant and upsetting experience that was likely to increase the adoptive mother's anxiety. In this family, too, the adopters were unwilling to risk an interview for the son after having had this threatening experience many years ago.

In a case mentioned earlier in this chapter the birth mother soon after the placement had taken the adoptive mother to her own home for convalescence from an illness. Some years later, while on holiday, the adoptive family passed through the area where they knew the birth mother had lived and they believe they saw her working as a sales assistant in a store. The adoptive mother commented to the child, then 8 or 9 years old, saying who this person was, but the woman showed no sign of recognition. Whether this was actually the mother is uncertain, but it seems that the adoptive mother would have been glad to renew the contact. This view is further supported by the fact that when the birth mother approached the girl through a mutual acquaintance just a few months before our interview and asked to see her, the adoptive mother was pleased rather than annoyed or fearful and thought her daughter should comply with the request. This she did without much enthusiasm.

There were six cases in which the birth mother visited the adoptive home after the legal adoption, but only one of these visits was without prior arrangement with the family. In this case the adoptive father had found this young mother a job locally and she popped in unannounced soon after the adoption just as she had done before it. The others apparently had not fully understood the meaning of adoption and continued to visit as before, writing and saying when to expect them. One brought her new husband to see the child before they emigrated, and a second continued to visit even after she married, but the adopters asked her to discontinue visiting when they learned that her husband did not know about the child. A third mother visited for three or four years after the adoption, then tapered off. In a fourth case the adopters felt it was 'quite a shock' when the mother wrote soon after the adoption that she would visit. She did so only twice, but continued to correspond with the adoptive mother until the child was 6 years old and the contact was ended then at the adoptive mother's request. In the fifth case the birth mother had died and the grandmother kept in touch with visits and letters to the adopters until the boy was in his teens. The grandmother then stepped out of the picture, as she felt it would be awkward for the boy when he realised who she really was.

In the strangest situation of all an adoptive father had made a serious effort to locate his son's birth mother to learn if she had other children as they would be this boy's half-siblings. Because of the boy's nationality background, which was the same as the adopters', the father felt he should be able to trace the mother among the small group of these people in Britain. This was a doting, over-protective family who had tried to give the boy everything and said they now wanted to give him brothers or sisters as well – but only if they were found to be suitable companions for the boy. In addition, and this was probably the basic cause for the search, the adoptive mother feared that in their small ethnic community the boy might meet and marry a half-sister without being aware of the blood relationship. The father found a woman he was convinced was the natural mother, but she emphatically denied any knowledge of the boy, much less having given birth to him. She had children whom the adoptive father was told were 'a poor sort', so he did not tell his son about them though he sometimes hints to the boy that he has knowledge of his background which he has not told him.

As might be expected, when a child was adopted by his foster parents there was more often contact between adoptive parents and the child's natural mother in the years after legal adoption than there was in cases where the child was adopted directly. In many foster parent adoptions this was a continuation and tapering-off of a relationship with the adopters, as well as with the child, and usually was not associated with the trauma and panic that anxious adopters, and more often fiction and the media, would have us believe are likely to accompany such contacts.

It may be of interest that in the families mentioned above, where there was personal contact between the adopters and some member of the child's birth family after the formalities of legal adoption had taken place, this did not appear to have caused difficulties for the adoptees. Of the six who were available for interview, five were rated as making a good or excellent current adjustment and one a marginal adjustment. The two who were not seen were described by their parents as happy and getting along well.

Chapter 9

◆

TALKING ABOUT ADOPTION

Communication within the family about adoption is considered by professionals as a crucial issue and Margaret Kornitzer, probably quite rightly, has said it is the 'telling' that proves the adoption. This is because of the tests that 'telling' poses to the adoptive parents' security in their role, to their sensitivity to their child's questions and his need for information or reassurance and to their own capacity to accept and empathise with his background.

Experience gained from the very early adoption placements of the 1930s and 1940s showed the damage that could be done by late and inept 'telling'. There were many stories of adolescent children being estranged from their adoptive parents, running away from home or showing other signs of distress caused by the shock of suddenly learning of their adoptive status. So, when the adoptees in this study were being placed at the end of the 1940s and the early 1950s, agencies already were urging adopters to tell their children very early, certainly before starting school, in order to avoid the knowledge being brought to them in an unpleasant or traumatic way. However, at that time social workers were primarily concerned that the child should know he was adopted and wanted. They were not much concerned with identity and had not fully appreciated the complexity of the task they were urging the new parents to undertake. As the Glasgow child psychiatrist Dr Fred Stone pointed out in 1969, the adopters are put in a double bind when they accept the child as their own and encourage him to feel he is theirs, yet tell him he is not. The adopters' problems with this and the resulting failures in communication were only too clearly revealed in the interviews in this current study.

Looking back now at the advice and information given by social workers and at the attitudes of the adopters, it is easy to feel censorious and point out the inadequacies, but the events must be seen in the context of the times if they are to be understood properly. The social climate in the late 1940s and early 1950s was different in many respects from that of the late 1970s when this is being written, particularly with regard to some key issues in adoption, such as illegitimacy and heredity. One has to remember that to most people at that time illegitimacy was shameful – a real stigma. This undoubtedly lay behind the emphasis on confidentiality carried to such lengths of secrecy and sometimes deceit. Agencies were concerned to protect the unmarried mother's guilty secret and adopters sought to protect their child from painful taunts or feelings of shame over his origins.

At that time emphasis was on the 'fresh start' provided by adoption and little thought was given to the child's need to know something of his biological heritage. Even in social work circles, it was not yet generally accepted that knowledge of origins was an important part of developing a balanced and mature sense of identity. The hope was that the adopted child or the child in care would 'forget' early painful experiences and just accept his present good home. Notions of genealogical bewilderment and complexities of identity for the adopted person were not raised until writers such as Sants (1964), Stone (1969) and Triseliotis (1973 and 1974) helped to elucidate them and brought them to people's attention.

The use of the expression 'telling' is itself significant. The impression was given that it would be sufficient to tell the child the fact that he was adopted and that the subject could then be closed. Little was done to alert adopters to the need for a series of discussions according to the child's age and capacity to understand and absorb the information. They were advised to 'tell' the child early, and a fairy story or tale of a baby found in the woods was quite often suggested as suitable, but very little help was given over how to deal with the difficult questions that the child might ask or indeed about the importance of enabling him to ask questions. Rather naturally it was assumed that when a child was ready for more information he would ask for it as he would about other subjects. It was only when McWhinnie's study of adopted adults was published in 1966 that it was realised that the adopters' discomfort with the subject would be communicated to the children to such a degree that they would be unable to ask questions, that in these circumstances the more loyal and loving the child, the fewer questions he would be likely to ask. These findings were fully supported by the accounts of 'telling' given by the families in the present project.

TIMING THE TELLING

When adopters were asked the age at which their child was first told they had adopted him and that he had once had other parents, nearly three in four told us that the child knew before he was 5 years old; they had made sure they had told him before he went to school. Nearly all the other children were reported to have learned it between the ages of 5 and 10. Only two children were said to have learned it later, one at 11 and the other at 14, although later, when we saw the adoptees themselves, 11 of that smaller group could not recall knowing it until they were more than 10 years old. It seems that some parents told the child as a toddler and did not mention it again; the child apparently accepted it as just another bed-time story and did not remember it. Reluctance to upset a child or their relationship with him may have caused other parents to touch upon the matter so lightly that it made no impression at all on the young child. Jaffee (1974) also found in his study of grown-up adoptees that, although in general their views were in agreement with their parents on other important subjects, they were in striking disagreement on the way their adoptive status had been presented and subsequently dealt with. Jaffee went on to point out the pivotal role that revelation and subsequent handling of the subject of adoption may play in the adoptee's self-concept and psychosocial health and in the quality of his relationship with his adoptive parents.

There were four adoptees whose parents believed they had *never* learned of their adoption. Two of these were foster parent adoptions and two were direct adoptions. One family had not told their son because he was too severely mentally handicapped to be able to understand, but there seemed to be no obvious reason to explain why the three other families had never told their daughters. The father of one of these girls explained it simply by saying: 'It would have upset her and it would have done no good to anyone.'

Oddly, late revelation of the fact that these were not birth parents occurred more frequently among the foster parent adoptions than among direct adoptions. Even when a birth mother was visiting in the foster home this was often done without the child's knowledge of the relationship. This may have been because it is even harder to explain relationships when a child's future is still uncertain.

Five children had experienced a period of doubt or uncertainty before actually learning that these were not their birth parents and, of these, four were first placed for fostering. A girl who was very different from her family had always wondered why, and she found it a relief to know that she was 'adopted and chosen'. A boy had overheard his mother say she couldn't have children, so he wondered how she had him. Three other children wondered why the 'lady from the orphanage' came to see them and why their surnames were different from other children in the family. Some of these youngsters had felt a nagging doubt about their identity for as long as three or more years before learning the truth.

When explanations were postponed they also were more likely to be given in a far from ideal context and to cause the child distress. For reasons unknown, older children who had the truth about their origins revealed under unfavourable circumstances were nearly all boys. None of them first learned of his adoption by finding documents or other papers or in connection with dating or marriage as is so often portrayed in fiction. Over 90 per cent of the children were said to have heard about their adoption from the parents themselves, usually from the adoptive mother or both parents together, but all too often those who were 5 years of age or older had learned it from someone else. Fathers alone seldom took responsibility for this task, and indeed several fathers said they felt telling was a mother's duty! Like those in McWhinnie's study, the adoptees were emphatic that the source of such important information should be their parents and not outsiders. There were two families whose children had had fairly serious personality problems who blamed these on 'early telling', though in one of these cases the boy, legally adopted at 12, had actually not been told of his foster status until after he went to school.

An example of damaging revelation came from parents who reported telling their son at 11 when he had been caught taking coins from his mother's purse. The mother had been unhappy with the adoption almost from the start and she took this opportunity to tell the boy how she really felt, saying: 'I'm not your mummy, Daddy is not your daddy and Sis is not your sister. We picked you out from a lot of babies and now you let us down.' These parents were unwilling for us to interview their son but they described him as having been an unhappy and rebellious adolescent who had been taken into care at their request.

Another boy, whose mother said he had learned at 14, was told by her after relatives visiting in the home had been overheard discussing him, while yet another little boy was told of his foster status at 6 years of age on the insistence of the social worker. In this case the birth mother was in the habit of visiting regularly and she had complained to the social worker that the boy called the foster mother 'Mummy'. Next time the mother visited, the foster mother told the child against her own better judgement and casually with the tea-towel in her hand. The little boy came in from play, saying, 'Mummy can I have an ice cream?' She said, 'I'm not your mummy'. He looked at her blankly and she went on, 'No, honestly, I'm not. Aunt Josie is really your mummy'. Unbelieving, the child came up and pulled at her skirt and said, 'You *are* my mummy'. She said, 'No, I'm not, Love, there is your mummy'. The little boy ran out of the house and into the garden screaming, 'You *are so* my mummy'. The foster mother turned to the birth mother and said: 'There, I told him.'

An example of another kind of late telling came from a family where the adoptive mother gave details of the rather involved story she had told her son more than once when he was a young child, but apparently he had never understood that it applied to him. He told us it came as a shock to him when at the age of 12 or 13 he overheard his mother and a friend talking about adoption and his name came into it. He never felt able to tell his mother what he had overheard, so there had been no communication between them about the adoption, and the mother continued to think that the son had known since a small child and that he had no problem about it. This unhappy and maladjusted young man said the fact that he had 'no history and nothing to relate to' now hangs over him 'like a great black cloud that overshadows everything else'.

When the adopted people in the study learned by the time they were 5 years old, they were usually told a story which was a mixture of fact and fiction and which they liked to hear over and over again. Those who were under 5 when they were told mostly received the news with pride or pleasure or sometimes with indifference; it was only among the older children that parents had noticed any sign of shock or bitterness (Table 9.1). Telling before 5 years of age definitely appears to have been the least damaging even though many did not really understand the significance of the story until much later.

Table 9.1   *Adoptees' reaction to first knowledge of their adoption, related to age at disclosure*

	Age at disclosure							
	Under 5 years		5 years or older		Never told		Total	
	no.	%	no.	%	no.	%	no.	%
Reaction								
Pride, pleasure	43	37	7	18	—	—	50	31
Indifference	58	49	19	49	—	—	77	48
None (child too young)	15	13	—	—	—	—	15	9
Stunned, shocked or bitter	—	—	6	15	—	—	6	4
Reaction unknown to parents	—	—	5	13	—	—	5	3
Not covered	1	1	2	5	4	100	7	5
Total	117	100	39	100	4	100	160	100

Thus, contrary to the views of two or three American psychiatrists (Schecter, 1960: Peller, 1961), who believe from child guidance work that it is less harmful to tell the child during the latency period than to tell him earlier before he has resolved the Oedipal phase, experience in this study tends to support the advice given to adoptive parents by social workers over the years – to tell the child early before someone else does. It also supports Triseliotis's research findings (1974, p.155) that 'those who found out late or came to know about their adoption from outside sources were the most hurt and upset'.

SHARING INFORMATION

Having nerved themselves to explain to the child that they were his adoptive parents, the parents then had to make decisions about how much information about his background should be shared. Of course, the adopters' ability to provide this information depended on what they themselves knew – often not very much — but as the interviews went on the project staff were increasingly concerned about the extent to which basic background data had been withheld, distorted or forgotten.

Only one in four of the adopted persons who were interviewed remembered ever being told the following basic facts: why they had been relinquished for adoption; when and where they were adopted, including the name of the agency and why the adopters took them; the personal and social characteristics of their biological parents. The others said they had been given only bits of this information and one in five had received virtually nothing beyond the fact of adoption.

Even when parents did pass on to the adopted children everything they knew about the child's first family, this information did not necessarily include all the points mentioned above, as some families said their agency had told them almost nothing about the biological family. In the case records of nearly all the direct adoptions there was a copy of a short letter which had been sent to adopters at the time the child was offered to them. This described the baby and such details of the parents as age and occupation, sometimes also education, social class and the reasons why the child was offered for adoption. These letters, brief as they were, were often 'forgotten' by the adopters. In the cases of the former foster children there was very seldom any record of what information had been given. Presumably the placement worker used her discretion about what information to give verbally at the time of placement or on later visits to the home. Presumably, too, the natural mother visiting in many of these homes may have added first-hand information. Certainly, foster parents who had become adoptive parents to the child were much better than direct adopters about sharing what they knew about him although they sometimes did this very late.

Overall, there was a definite tendency for parents not to divulge all they knew about the children's background and the circumstances of their birth and placement. Less than 40 per cent of the parents said they had given their child all the information they themselves knew. Jaffee and Fanshel (1970, p.312) found only 12 per cent of the adopters in their study had shared with their children the true facts of the adoption as they knew them. More than 25 per cent in our study had omitted or falsified some of the facts and another 30 per cent had revealed the child's adoptive status but had given him no information at all about his background. As we have already seen, four parents had withheld even the bare fact of adoption. Oddly, quite a few parents reported that the only information they had given the child about his background was the fact of his illegitimacy. Perhaps they felt the child would recognise his illegitimate birth as the most acceptable reason for being given up for adoption. But to give this one unpalatable bit of information alone also suggests its importance to the adopters and in some families, at least, a need to punish the child for something they themselves had never been able to accept.

Something else that the project staff noticed again and again was that parents frequently withheld the kind of background information which would have been reassuring to their adopted children. For instance, when they had met the birth mother and could have satisfied the child's wish to know what she looked like, they failed to mention the meeting. Nor did they usually let the child know the mother had found the decision for adoption a difficult one. When this was mentioned at all it was likely to be in terms of the mother holding up the adoption. In cases where the biological family had traits or occupations which would have raised the adopted person's self-esteem this information more often than not was withheld. Examples of this were a girl who became a nurse and unknown to her the biological mother had also been a SRN, and a boy who studied surveying but had never been told that members of his birth family had been chartered surveyors. Perhaps if the adopted people had asked direct questions about these things more parents would have disclosed them, but children did not often do this for, as we have seen, they did not feel comfortable about it.

Some parents (nearly one in three) wished they had known more about their child's background, seeing it as a possible explanation for something in the child's development or personality which they had not understood, but a smaller number knew something they wished they had never been told. More than one in five found that some of the information they had been given was an obstacle to communication with the child about his background. There were other parents who had worried that something important was withheld from them by the agency and this, too, made discussion harder. In all, nearly one-third had been worried about something, either known or unknown to them, in the child's background and it was most often the less satisfied parents who had these worries.

The interviewers were also impressed by how often people ignored even the few facts given them and imagined a background that fitted their idea of what the heritage of an adopted child, and of this one in particular, should be. For example, there was a woman with a stereotype of unmarried mothers, who always feared her attractive daughter would have an illegitimate baby at an early age 'like her young unmarried mother', whereas she had been told at the time of placement that the girl's natural mother was not young or unmarried, but instead was over 30 when this child was born and was a married woman who had had several children of the marriage.

Imagination also ran riot when parents had been given no information or had been told the agency did not have the facts, such as information about the child's putative father or the social class of his birth mother. In these circumstances adopters tended to grasp at straws. For example, a mother hearing her 8 year-old gleefully mimic the cries of vendors in a market wondered if his first father had been a street trader, and a middle-class family decided their son's background must be working class because of his enthusiasm for candyfloss.

In general there appeared to be a great deal of very confused thinking even among well-educated people about what traits can and cannot be inherited. Concern about heredity was ever present in some families to the extent that nurture hardly had a chance, and in others (probably in most) it seemed to lurk just below the surface to appear when problems arose.

FREQUENCY OF DISCUSSION

How often was the subject of adoption mentioned between parents and children over the years? Were they comfortable in discussing it after the hurdle of the first revelation had been overcome? Were the adopted persons satisfied with what they had been given?

As already noted, there seems to have been a serious breakdown in communication between parents and children on this subject, with the result that some adoptees who had been told when very young did not fully understand until they were much older, sometimes not until adolescence.

It certainly can be said that most of these families did not discuss the matter often. The largest number of parents, nearly half, said it was spoken of only two or three times over the years, and another quarter perhaps as often as once or twice a year. Four families mentioned it as often as once a month but seven other families (4 per cent) never mentioned it again after the first telling. These last often said that they assumed the child had accepted it and possibly 'forgotten'. However, they may not have been very confident of this, since (along with those who had never told the child at all) these were the parents who were most often unwilling for their son or daughter to take part in the research. There were also those who had never been able to face the child with the facts. They had made no secret of the adoption and had discussed it openly between themselves or with others while the child was present, or they had left correspondence and Christmas cards from the adoption agency lying about the house, but they had never told the child outright or discussed it with him directly.

It will be recalled that not much relationship was found between the adoptees' adjustment and how often adoption had been discussed, but Jaffee and Fanshel (1970, p.268) found that the more frequently reference was made to the adoptee's status over the years, the more likely he was to encounter adjustment problems while growing up. Fanshel's finding seems to say that even a good thing can be carried too far or done insensitively or for the wrong reasons. In fact one of the few families in the current study who had mentioned adoption very frequently actually did this when they were displeased with the child to remind him of the inevitability of a tragic life ahead because of his heredity (actually not very bad) and his illegitimate birth. Another who mentioned it very often had still given the child very little information. It seems that parental attitudes towards the subject of adoption and background are likely to be more important than the amount of information disclosed or the frequency with which the subject is raised, though these attitudes are harder to measure.

Fewer than a third of the families said they had felt comfortable in talking with their children about background, and this showed no relationship to social class even though middle-class families are usually considered to be more verbal. The interviewers assessing the parents' present ease with the subject felt that even now in this interview and without the adoptee present, more than half were still uncomfortable and wished to avoid it or at least skip over the subject lightly.

This degree of discomfort with the subject that is at the very core of the adoption experience is disquieting but not unusual. As we have seen, other investigators too have found a general reluctance among adoptive parents to share information about the child's genealogy and how he came to be adopted.

This problem is often thought to be associated with unresolved conflict over infertility. The parents in this study almost certainly had had no help in coming to terms with this, as it was never once mentioned in the case records. However, feelings about infertility and childlessness are not the only reason for adopters' discomfort with the subject of their child's first family. Some of the people in the study had biological as well as adopted children, and yet they found it very difficult to discuss the adopted child's background with him. It seems that a negative attitude to illegitimacy and questions about their own right to parent the child (perhaps arising from conflict about infertility), as well as fear of losing his love, were additional problems which entered into the parents' discomfort. In some cases it seemed that adopters believed that any mention of the child's natural family would subject them to competition with that other family for the child's love and loyalty.

Nor was it only the parents who found it hard to talk. When the adoptees were asked whether they felt they could ask for more information if they wanted it, just over half had not felt free to raise the subject with their parents, although they discussed it apparently quite comfortably with the interviewer. They realised it was a very sensitive subject and did not wish to hurt, anger or antagonise their parents by referring to it. The difficulties adoptees felt in bringing up the subject are illustrated by a young man who said his mother 'always gets tearful when adoption is mentioned on television' and a young woman who said her family speak of it in hushed tones 'as if there were a death in the house'. However, there was also considerable anxiety among the adoptees about what the information on birth parents might be like if they got it, and it seemed that this worry, too, might lie behind the hesitation in seeking information. So the adopted people were just as often as their adoptive parents uncomfortable in communicating with each other on this vital topic, and this included some whose overall adjustment was excellent.

Much the same picture emerges from Leeding's survey (1977) of adopted adults who had taken advantage of the Children Act, 1975, to get some information from their original birth records. Most of those adoptees were keeping the search secret from their parents, a frequent comment being: 'It would hurt them too much if they knew.' Leeding points out that 'protection against the truth is a weapon which once used against the adopted child, now turns itself against the adopters in later life'.

It is interesting that by no means all the adoptees wanted further information. However, it could be that the project was denied access to those most wanting it, as despite assurances there was fear among parents that the interviewer might disclose something to the adoptee that would make him unsettled or turn his interest in the direction of his first parents.

The young people we saw were divided about evenly into thirds on this matter of the wish for additional information about their background. One-third were very contented with what they had been given, even when this was very little or nothing, another third were reasonably contented though they would have welcomed a little more information and the remaining third were rather dissatisfied with the information they had received or definitely wished for more (Table 9.2). Those who wished for more usually did not want a great deal of information but there were just one or two things they longed to know. Most often this was a desire to know the reason behind their being given for adoption or what their birth mother had looked like (especially when their own appearance was very different from the adopted family and they wondered whom they resembled).

Table 9.2   *Adoptees' contentment with background information given by adoptive parents*

	no.	%
Very contented	34	32
Reasonably contented but wished for a little more	31	30
Rather discontented	23	22 } 35
Very discontented, wished for much more	14	13 }
Not covered	3	3
Total	105	100

ATTITUDE TO BIRTH PARENTS

As we have already seen in Chapter 6 there was a close relationship between parental acceptance of birth parents and an adoptee's overall satisfaction with his adoption experience. However, many adopters had kept their feelings to themselves and virtually half the adoptees interviewed did not know how their adoptive parents felt about their birth parents. This was particularly true in direct adoption where two-thirds did not know and showed no anxiety about it. The former foster children much more often knew whether their adopters felt warmly towards the biological mother or were critical and disapproved of her. In these cases the first mother had been known to the adopters as the person who had approved of them as new parents for the child or had been a serious threat if she did not come quickly to a decision for adoption. Nearly a quarter of the former foster children believed their adoptive parents tended to disapprove of the birth parents.

As for the adoptees themselves, nearly three in four of the 105 who were interviewed were largely unconcerned with regard to their birth parents or else were understanding but felt no need to contact them. These adoptees seem to have become fully integrated into and identified with their adoptive families. Only four showed any interest in establishing a relationship with birth parents, but there were nineteen who said they would like to communicate with one or both just once or see them once, though they had never made any attempt to do so. Several of these had found themselves with an awakened interest in their biological parents at the time when they were marrying or having their first child. Others had been interested in adolescence but not afterwards. There were seven others who were rejecting and hostile towards their first parents, feeling abandoned by them, and they said they did not want any contact, though one might suspect some ambivalence about this. Four of these seven had first learned of their adoption when they were more than 5 years old. One wanted to tell his first mother what he thought of her and another bitter young man threatened to harm his mother if he should meet her (Table 9.3).

Table 9.3   *Adoptees' attitude to contacting birth parents*

	no.	%
Largely unconcerned, no wish for contact	53	50 ⎱ 71
Understanding but no wish for contact	22	21 ⎰
Rejecting or hostile, no wish for contact	7	7
Wish for one or more contacts	23	22
Total	105	100

Interest in contact with birth parents was related to the kind of care the adoptees felt they had received from the adoptive parents. They less often had any interest in seeing their birth parents when they had received plenty of love and affection from both adoptive parents. As we have already seen, it tended to be the less well-adjusted and less satisfied adoptees who were interested in getting in touch with birth parents. This corresponds with what Triseliotis found in Scotland and Fanshel found in the United States.

Two girls were interviewed who had a really deep desire to meet and establish an on-going relationship with their first mothers. They are interesting examples of adoptees still seeking for security and affection they have never had or have now lost. One of the two girls who very much wanted to know her birth mother had presented many problems while growing up and was still very anxious and pessimistic. She felt the adoptive mother had never been a proper mother to her and they were now estranged. Not surprisingly this girl cherished the idea that her birth mother would surely be a more caring person. The other girl was longing for a close relationship with her birth mother and had done so since she lost her adoptive mother several years ago. As she was unhappy in her marriage and felt unwelcome in the parental home since her father's remarriage, she was now keen to meet her other parents, but also too frightened to try. She had been daydreaming of a lasting and affectionate relationship with them and sometimes feared they might die before she could meet them, but she also feared that a meeting might shatter her fantasies. She said: 'It might be horrible; they might be living in a mud hut or something.' These young women were interviewed before the Children Act 1975, and one wonders if by now they have taken advantage of the provision which allows access to birth records.

The only adoptee in the study who had already made a real effort to find his natural family was a young man who was not interviewed because his whereabouts were unknown. We know that at 15 he contacted social agencies and community leaders in a really desperate effort to trace his mother. He had never become reconciled to his adoptive mother leaving the family when he was 8, or the divorce that followed. Unfortunately, it is not known whether he found his biological mother. His only contact with his adoptive father is an occasional telephone call.

Among the adoptees whose parents were not willing for them to be interviewed were a few who, usually during adolescent rebellion, had threatened parents with finding their other parents. This was very effective against adopters who were insecure about full entitlement and sometimes it was quite effective in destroying parental discipline. There were also three who were said to have gone to Somerset House in London, where birth records were then kept, and three others had been in touch with their placement agency. Two of these would have liked to meet their birth parents but the others were said only to be seeking further information about their origins.

Two adoptees had already had a recent meeting with their birth mothers, but these were not the ones who had threatened this and there was no problem involved in finding the mothers. Both had been adopted after several years in the family as foster children and the birth mothers' whereabouts had never been a secret. One of these has been mentioned in Chapter 8 – the girl whose birth mother had been very friendly with the adoptive mother when the girl was with the family on a fostering basis and the birth mother had recently intitiated a contact with her. This young woman felt rather neutral about the meeting and thought it might have had more meaning for this mother than for her. In the other case the young man knew where his birth mother lived, as he had gone there once with his foster mother before the legal adoption was completed. He called in to see her recently when his work took him to her village, and was surprised and hurt by the rather cool welcome he received at this unexpected visit. As we have seen, there was a third girl who at 16 had seen her birth mother, but this was for the purpose of getting her consent to this late adoption and therefore took place before the legalisation.

In summing up it must be said that many adoptive parents and children in the study had a great deal of difficulty in talking with each other about the child's background and adoptive status. Parents felt they could not keep the subject open without risk to the warm feeling of belonging which had developed between them and the child; children hesitated to raise questions as they sensed the pain this would cause to their parents and because of their own anxiety about the information they might learn about their backgrounds. It was freedom to raise the subject, not the frequency of discussion, that was important to adoptees. Hoping to avoid discussion, parents depended upon the children to raise questions if they wanted to know more than they had been told, but relatively few adoptees felt free to do this even now.

Chapter 10

———◆———

FAMILY RELATIONSHIPS

Adoption agencies have always tried their best to ensure that the babies they place have a happy and secure childhood. At first they concentrated most on material advantages, church affiliation and making sure that the child would be kindly treated. As experience grew, it became clear that by no means all those who might make adequate parents to children born to them would make satisfactory adopters. The emphasis shifted to motivation. Much stress was laid on the need for both husband and wife to be keen to adopt, on the dangers of adopted children being wanted only as companions, on problems arising from unresolved feelings of anguish over infertility. There was increasing recognition that adoptive families were not just the same as others, but it took a long time to reach a proper understanding of what their extra difficulties really were. As so often with these complex problems, in the end it came down to the deceptively simple but quite fundamental question of whether or not an adoptive family considered themselves to be a 'real' family with the right to parent the child, whether they had feelings of 'entitlement'. It is this basic issue which creates the extra dimension that separates adoptive from ordinary families (though step-parent families face some of the same questions). Entitlement encompasses an interlocking web of feelings about parenthood, self-worth, genealogy, heredity, fertility and some deep-seated attitudes towards giving and receiving.

THE CONCEPT OF ENTITLEMENT

Rosner (1961) wrote of the crisis of self-doubt that can afflict adoptive families, and Krugman (1964) described how a group of ordinary citizens was divided between those who thought real parents were always those who gave birth and those who thought that real parenthood was bringing children up. Rowe (1970) pointed out how general (even among social workers) is the distinction between 'own child' and 'adopted child' and emphasised the need for understanding of the special tasks to be accomplished in establishing a secure adoptive relationship. She pointed to the powerful weapon the adopted child can wield when he says 'I bet my real mother would let me do that' or 'I wish you had never adopted me'.

The confidence to deal with this kind of taunt, to exercise normal parental discipline and to be open about the facts of adoption without fear of losing the child's love, comes from a sense of entitlement to the child. Jaffee and Fanshel (1970, p. 14) coined this word to explain a concept which adoption workers had only partially recognised before. They say: 'We speculated that whatever hazards existed in adoption from the standpoint of parental behaviour, these were likely to stem from the parents' inability to feel that the adopted children truly belonged to them.' Jaffee and Fanshel felt they had not been able to prove their hypothesis about entitlement because the results of their complex analysis of the data they had collected about family functioning were inconclusive. They were also greatly hampered by their inability to interview more than a small proportion of the adoptees in the families they studied. This meant that in the other cases they had to rely on the parents' view of their child's adjustment to adult life and could get no first-hand information about the effect on the child of his parents' feeling of security or insecurity in their roles.

In our project we had the great advantage of being able to interview a substantial proportion of the adoptees. Though we, too, were convinced of the crucial importance of the concept of entitlement it proved elusive and difficult to demonstrate. The presence or absence of the feeling can only be gauged by inference. It is not something one can ask a direct question about or put into a statistical table. Its absence is reflected in parental anxiety over losing the child's affection, in over-protectiveness, in inability to answer questions about origins and in attitudes towards natural parents. Its presence manifests itself in a confident and robust approach to family relationships by both adopter and adoptee and about these it was possible to gather a considerable amount of information.

CLOSENESS OF PARENTS AND CHILD

The parents and young people were asked to look back over their relationship and comment on their closeness over the years. More than two-thirds of the parents but only half the young people assessed their relationship as close during all the years that the child was growing up in the family. (Another quarter of the adoptees had felt close to one of the parents but not the other.) In addition to those parents who had always had a close relationship with their child, there were others who had felt this way except during the child's adolescence, and still others who had enjoyed a close relationship at first but the child's adolescent rebellion had come between them to such an extent that the relationship had not recovered from it. There also were 11 sets of parents (7 per cent) in the total parent group of 160 who said they had never felt close to the child, and in the smaller group of 105 adoptees who were seen 15 said they had never felt close to either adoptive parent and 6 others thought they had been closer to a sibling or a grandparent.

The closeness a child felt to his adoptive parents over the years seemed to be unrelated to several factors which we had thought might be associated with it, namely, the child's sex, his age at this placement, earlier residential nursery care, the number of different living arrangements before coming to live with this family, or the basis on which he had been placed with them. One might think that girls more often than boys would have had a close relationship with their family, since so many studies have shown adopted boys presenting problems in growing up. Or, following Bowlby's theories, one might suppose that a period of residential nursery care as a baby, or several different caretaking arrangements before this permanent placement, might have made it impossible for children to relate warmly to adoptive parents, but this was not found to be so. One also wonders, when children have been received first on a fostering basis (often with a natural mother visiting in the home), whether the relationship between adoptive parents and child becomes as close as when children are taken specifically for adoption. This idea, like the others, was found to have no foundation in fact (Table 10.1).

Table 10.1 *Feeling of closeness to adoptive parents over the years, related to basis on which adoptees were received into their families*

	Basis on which child was received into family							
	Adoption only		Fostering with a view to adoption		Fostering only		Total	
	no.	%	no.	%	no.	%	no.	%
Feeling of closeness								
Close to both parents	28	57	22	49	6	55	56	53
Mostly close to mother	5	10	9	20	3	27	17	16
Mostly close to father	4	8	4	9	1	9	9	9
Close to someone else	3	6	2	4	1	9	6	6
Close to no one	9	19	6	13	—	—	15	14
Not covered	—	—	2	5	—	—	2	2
Total	49	100	45	100	11	100	105	100

Combining young children and families with the hope of achieving close and affectionate bonds is no small task for adoption agencies because loving relationships result from an interaction of needs, experiences and temperaments which modify each other and which cannot always be predicted. In the study we saw families where parents had responded very differently to individual children and had handled them in quite different ways, usually irrespective of which were their natural children and which were adopted. In some families, where parents and adopted children had never developed a really close relationship, the interviewer felt the child might well have done so in a different family and that these parents could have responded more warmly to a child of different temperament.

Believing that the atmosphere in the homes while the children were growing up there must have had its effect upon them, we tried to assess this atmosphere from what we knew of the families in the early case records and in the research interviews. This was, of course, very subjective, but as it was feeling tones which were being evaluated these could in any event hardly be otherwise. As a result of this assessment, half the homes were considered to have provided the child in the study with an atmosphere of well-being and security, of warm and harmonious relationships throughout the whole of childhood. Another third were able to provide this for some of the time, but in these families the climate had deteriorated over the years. In the remainder of the homes – 28 in all – there was anxiety, insecurity or conflict during a large part of the subjects' childhood.

Changes in family climate, of course, are frequently unpredictable and have many different causes, among them: the death of a parent coming either as a sudden shock or following a long illness; marital disharmony with or without separation or divorce; problems with other children in the family or with relatives; personality changes over the years; and not least the family's reaction to the developing child, especially if they lack commitment, are disappointed in him or frustrated in efforts to mould him to their ways. Some adoptees survived family calamities well, when these came fairly late in childhood after a long period of warm and secure relationships within the home. In the few cases where they struck earlier, or no really warm and satisfying relationship had existed almost from the beginning of the placement, the adoptees had suffered acutely over the years.

Although an abundance of love and caring was the dominant recollection of the great majority of adoptees, this generally cheerful picture has to be set against those cases – few in number but vivid in detail – where things had not been so happy.

One young man, mentioned earlier because he was very dissatisfied with his adoption, felt he had been subjected to abuse and neglect. He illustrated this by saying that when his mother was in hospital his father used to visit her, leaving the son at home to do the chores. Feeling sorry for himself with work to do when other youngsters were free to play, and perhaps anxious about his mother and feeling left out, he said he got into 'lots of trouble' for which his father 'beat' him. After a very rebellious adolescence this man has now married and is supporting his family, but in our opinion his adjustment appears precarious. Although this was the only adoptee among those interviewed who felt he had ever been physically abused or neglected, one woman said she and also the natural-born child in her home had been 'terrified' of their mother whom she described as 'a big woman with a bad temper'.

There was more than one example of a child finding life in the adoptive family very difficult after one loving parent had died, especially if the remaining parent had remarried and there were step-brothers or sisters. And among the parents who were unwilling for their son or daughter to take part in the study we came across a family where the mother became quite hysterical and abusive when the interviewer inquired about seeing the son. This young man had been rejected throughout his childhood, had often run away from home and his mother now had nothing good to say for him. The interviewer wondered if the parents were afraid of what the son might say about his adoption if he were interviewed.

THE ADOPTED CHILD'S PLACE IN THE FAMILY

We have already seen that adoptees were more likely to be making a good adjustment, as well as being more satisfied, when parents described the relationships within the family as well balanced, than in households where life had revolved around this child or else he had been treated as somehow 'inferior'. Being the centre of attention was no more helpful than holding a rather low status, perhaps because neither would help an adopted child to feel he belonged in the family.

Table 10.2 *Adoptees' status in the family, related to their feeling of likeness to parents*

	Feeling of likeness to parents							
	Like or somewhat like		Unlike or uncertain		Not covered		Total	
	no.	%	no.	%	no.	%	no.	%
Status in family								
As biological child	68	94	17	59	2	50	87	83
As foster or step-child or too 'special'	4	6	11	38	1	25	16	15
Not covered	—	—	1	3	1	25	2	2
Total	72	100	29	100	4	100	105	100

Eighty-seven of the adoptees who were seen felt they had been treated as a natural child of the family, but ten felt they had been more of a foster child or step-child; one of these referred to his adoptive mother as 'my step-mother' and another described the relationship in that way. Six said that although their parents had not treated them as though born to them, they had not been made to feel inferior; they had in fact been indulged and over-protected to an extent they believed would not happen with a biological child. These adoptees tended to attribute this over-indulgence to their adopters' persistent fear that they would want to return to their birth parents, or earlier that their birth parents might appear to reclaim them. In one case the adopted daughter (quiet, artistic and self-contained) was so different from her active and hearty family that they felt they could only leave her to develop in her own way. She was not guided or disciplined like the other children in the family and she now felt she could have used some guidance.

There was a definite association between feeling treated as a biological child of the family and feeling like the family in one way or another (Table 10.2). No doubt adopters find it easier to parent a child who is like them, but probably the children also begin to see likenesses when they are treated as though born to these parents, with the result that these feelings may be built up through interaction. Perhaps it might be expected, too, that being treated as a biological child would be associated with developing a sense of personal worth, and indeed three in four of those who felt they were treated like this were in fact considered to have a realistic sense of their own value, while this was true of less than one in five of the few who felt they were not treated in this way.

DECISIONS AND DISCIPLINE

Over half the parents said important decisions concerning the child had been made by both of them together and a few said the child had been included in such decisions. Somewhat fewer of the *adoptees* we were able to see thought the decisions had been made jointly by mother and father; more thought they had been made by their mother, and that this was as it should be.

More than half the parents considered they had been moderate in their control over the child in the study. Another one in five thought they had exercised only a minimum of restraint (perhaps too little, some thought now in retrospect), and one in seven believed they had been strict. A few parents were aware that their control had been inconsistent, in as much as one parent had been strict and the other lenient, or they had been too strict on some occasions and too easy-going at other times. As might be expected, the adoptees somewhat more often saw their parents as having been strict or inconsistent. However, it was interesting that those who felt their parents had been strict often qualified this (particularly if they now had children of their own) by saying they had recently come to a different view of the need for parental control and would like to bring up their children in the same way they themselves had been raised.

During the course of the study it became increasingly clear to the interviewers that parents who had little feeling of entitlement to their child – for whatever reason – were often incapable of disciplining him. Such people felt they had little right to the child, that in spite of the legal ties that bound them to him there were stronger ties which still bound him to his birth mother, and if they overstepped by denying him anything he wanted or by disciplining him in other ways he might withdraw his love for them and seek his other mother. This fear seemed to be far more prevalent than adoption workers realise and its consequences could be disastrous. Whereas most of the adoptees who felt their parents had exerted moderate and consistent control over them were now well-adjusted young adults, this was the situation with only half who felt their parents had been too lenient, inconsistent or contradictory.

As we have seen, adoptees welcomed some freedom to follow their own interests, to take some risks and choose their own friends and career. They resented parents who were possessive or overprotective and who discouraged or did not let them follow their own interests.

One in eight said he had been held back in this way and it was noticeable that this happened much more often when the adoptive mother had been over 40 when the child was placed. Two in three had felt free to make their own choices about important issues such as training and careers, though in a few families only one parent had been sympathetic to the adoptee's wish to decide these things for himself.

There were as many as one in five young people who considered one or both of their parents (most often the mother) as possessive or overprotective and the interviewers saw a few families where this was very evident even to an outsider. For example, a young man already mentioned because of his poor overall adjustment was still accompanied by his mother whenever he went into town, and when he accepted her decision that he should change his job she went along with him to the interview. More than one young man had recently married and was struggling to free himself from a loving but possessive mother, and the mother of a boy not yet married was proud of the 'dutiful' son who, she said, never goes out with people his age but only with her.

CURRENT PARENT-CHILD RELATIONSHIPS

Four-fifths of the total group of parents and a similar proportion of the young adults considered their present relationship to be warm and satisfying, though the latter sometimes thought their relationship was warmer with one parent (usually the mother) than with the other. We do not know how these figures compare with non-adopted families, but at a time of rapid social change, when many parents and young people are finding it particularly difficult to bridge the generation gap, it seems rather encouraging that more than three out of four adoptees still felt close to their families, and even a slightly larger proportion of parents still had a warm and satisfying relationship with their child.

In two-thirds of the families the parents' predominant feeling towards these children now appeared to be pleasure and pride, and nearly half could now recall no serious anxieties or tensions in their relationship. As they talked about the child, it was affection, pride and understanding which were most often clearly revealed. Many were very much enjoying helping the young people establish a home, welcoming sons- or daughters-in-law into the family and especially welcoming the grandchildren. Only in six families (4 per cent) were the parents now clearly rejecting or indifferent to the adoptee, though a few other parents were worried or anxious and there were twenty-eight – getting on for one in five – who seemed primarily disappointed or hurt, and in eight families the mother and father now showed strikingly different feelings for the child.

Hurt and disappointment were shown equally in relation to sons and daughters, but worry and anxiety were directed very much more often towards sons. One wonders if girls might have caused anxiety and worry earlier before they had married and settled down. Certainly, as we shall see in the chapter concerned with problems in growing up, a few of the girls had been very difficult in adolescence.

There was a clear association between the adoptees' current marital status and the closeness of the families' present relationships. Those adoptees who were married were more apt than those who were single or divorced to have a warm but adult relationship with their parents. Single adoptees, when the relationship was described as close, more often had a dependent relationship while those who were divorced usually had no close relationship at all with their parents. Perhaps those who were married had put their adolescent rebellion behind them and could now relate more positively to their parents, while some of those who were still single or who had tried marriage and failed might still be feeling rebellious and struggling for independence. Possibly in some other cases, too, parents were able to relax and enjoy their children more after the children were married and 'launched'.

'REAL' PARENTS AND 'OWN' CHILDREN

One of the most important and revealing questions which we put to the adoptees was about which set of parents they considered to be the 'real' ones. Did they think that 'it is the people who bring you up who really matter' or did they believe that 'blood is thicker than water', or were they confused about it?

The term 'real mother' is used so widely to mean the birth mother that some adoptees used it in this way, but when asked which parents they felt were the 'real' ones 81 per cent of the men and 89 per cent of the women said with no hesitation that it was the adoptive parents, the only ones they had known as parents. Fourteen were undecided or felt they had no real parents, but only one believed it definitely was the birth parents, and this was a girl who had been given good physical care but felt unloved.

Most striking was the association between feeling satisfied with the adoption experience and considering the adopters as the real parents. All but two of the eighty-three well-satisfied adoptees who were interviewed had no doubts on this score, and those two adoptees felt torn between the rival sets of parents. The adoptees who were less satisfied were much less sure, and none of the three who were very unhappy with their experience looked on the adopters as his real parents. Not surprisingly, those who had received plenty of affection and been treated as a natural child of the family responded with reciprocal feelings, while those who felt they had been given good physical care but not much love were divided in their loyalties. It seems clear that most had a mental image of how parents should behave and when adopters measured up to this they were seen as the real parents; when they did not, the adoptees felt uncertain and confused.

Some parents told us directly, others indirectly, whether they now looked upon the adoptee as their own son or daughter. Two-thirds of those with a son and three-quarters with a daughter had always felt the child was their own or very largely so, but in the little group of fourteen families who had taken the children just for fostering and had later adopted them, only seven now saw them as their own. Apparently it was not because legal adoption had been delayed for several years that these foster parent adopters felt the children did not truly belong, as legalisation was just as often late among the seven who felt the children were their own. Nor were these more often children who were older when placed with their families. Possibly the original intention, whether to foster or adopt, may have affected the parents' feeling of 'ownness' over the years.

Neither the adoptee's ordinal place in the family nor the presence or absence of younger brothers or sisters, whether natural or adopted, showed any apparent association with the adopters' feeling this was their child. However, their attitude to heredity seemed to be a factor which definitely was related to this. We found that only a little over 35 per cent of the people who had expected their child's future to be determined largely by the forces of heredity now felt the adoptee was their child; this was true of nearly 90 per cent of parents who had believed that the kind of life they provided for the child would largely determine the outcome, and more than 75 per cent of those who had attributed approximately equal influence to heredity and environment. Confidence in nurture was here once again demonstrated as an important factor in adoption outcome (Table 10.3).

A definite pattern can be seen linking the quality of the relationship which had existed between the parents and the adopted son or daughter throughout the years with the parents' feeling the child was their own. Nearly nine in every ten parents who had found their relationship with the child loving and enjoyable felt the child was their own, but fewer than three in five felt this way when life with the child had been difficult as well as loving, and even fewer felt the child was their own when they had been in constant conflict with him. Though the pattern is clear enough the meaning is more complex. At this late date it is impossible to make even approximate assessments of the extent to which the parents' uncertainties or lack of commitment led to the conflicts and behaviour problems or to know which came first, the difficulties or the distancing. Even in ordinary families, rather few parents attribute their children's bad behaviour to their own handling and it is not at all surprising that on an emotional level adopters sometimes 'disowned' their problem children.

There is also a cause and effect question about the relationship between the adopters' feeling the child as their own and their feeling he was like them in some respect. More than nine in ten of the parents who considered the child as very much like them also considered him as their own, whereas only one in five felt he was their own when they saw the child as very different. Even a small likeness apparently helped adopters to feel the child belonged in their family – or perhaps some parents began to see a likeness because they

Table 10.3 *Feeling adopted children their own, related to adoptive parents' attitude to influence of heredity and environment*

	Parents' attitude towards influence of heredity and environment							
	Greater reliance on heredity		Equal reliance on heredity and environment		Greater reliance on environment		Total	
	no.	%	no.	%	no.	%	no.	%
Adopters' feeling towards child								
Feel own child	15	36	49	77	48	89	112	70
Not sure	14	33	9	14	5	9	28	18
Not feel child is theirs	10	24	2	3	1	2	13	8
Incompatible responses	3	7	2	3	—	—	5	3
Not covered	—	—	2	3	—	—	2	1
Total	42	100	64	100	54	100	160	100

wanted so much to make the child their own. On the other hand it is bound to be difficult for parents to identify with a child whose personality they find uncongenial or whose behaviour they deplore. So perhaps it is almost inevitable that adopters whose children have serious problems of personality or behaviour tend to see them as different and find it difficult to acknowledge them as their own.

Chapter 11

———◆———

PROBLEMS IN GROWING UP

No account of the experiences of adoptive families could be considered complete without a detailed examination of the various difficulties they had faced in bringing up the children. Nevertheless there are particular problems about the material in this chapter which need to be pointed out by the writer and borne in mind by the reader.

The first is one that has been present throughout this book, but is particularly acute here, that is, that unusual families or those with problems are much more interesting than families or individuals who are ordinary and normal. There is really very little to say about healthy, happy people! Inevitably, therefore, in a book of this kind, more space is devoted to the minority of situations in which there were difficulties than to the straightforward, dull, but normal majority, and the illustrations are often drawn from the more extreme cases. This is especially true in a chapter devoted to a wide variety of problems many of which most families in the study never encountered.

Some figures are given in this chapter in order to offer a general idea about the proportion of cases in the project families in which certain problems occurred. But it must be stressed that these are based on the recollections of adoptive parents going back over more than 20 years and subject to error and the normal distortions of time. Therefore, no conclusions can be drawn about the proportion of children placed for adoption who would be likely to suffer from any of the conditions or display any of the behaviour characteristics described here. The case illustrations are quoted mainly for their intrinsic interest and not as typical examples except when this is specifically stated.

Finally, there is the difficulty noted in previous chapters, that there are almost no national figures or data from other studies which can be compared usefully with these findings. The problems described here occurred at some time during the whole childhood, adolescence and early adult years of the adoptees in this study. Other well-known studies such as that carried out on the Isle of Wight by Rutter *et al.*, (1970), the National Children's Bureau's child development study (Pringle *et al.*, 1966 and Fogelman, 1976) offered data on groups of children at particular stages in their development. The Isle of Wight study, for instance, was limited to children aged 10 and 11, so one cannot compare the incidence of problems in that population with their occurrence among adoptees. Published figures on delinquency rates are likewise of little help because they are concerned either with children and adolescents dealt with by juvenile courts or else with adults, and unfortunately we did not always obtain precise information on the age at which delinquent adoptees in our study committed their offences. So although we have a general picture of the incidence of problems in these families, we usually cannot say whether this is higher or lower than in the population at large.

We should also point out that this chapter will include in addition to behaviour and personality difficulties any problems of health or development which the parents reported.

HEALTH PROBLEMS

These days, health problems are seldom a serious impediment to adoption placement, as there are agencies now which specialise in finding families for children even if they have very serious handicaps. This was not so when the children in the project were being placed, and doctors were asked to examine the children to see whether they were 'fit for adoption', i.e. healthy enough to be offered to adopters. Sometimes a child was offered for adoption after a minor defect had been corrected, as happened with two of the adopted people in the study: one child had a harelip repaired and the other had club feet corrected before placement. A baby with a slight malformation of one hand was placed with no difficulty, but a child with a heart murmur was offered rather apologetically for fostering rather than adoption and described to the foster parents as 'not a perfect baby'.

Generally, therefore, adoptive parents during this era less often than ordinary parents found themselves bringing up a child with a congenital health problem. Among the children in the study there were, however, some instances of physical defects which were noted later, sometimes many years later. These include two children with poor eyesight, one with malformed legs which required surgery, and one with a 'genetic spinal condition' which affected his posture.

The children in the study had the usual childhood diseases, but one in seven also had a chronic or recurring medical condition, most often asthma, and another one in four had suffered from one or more serious illnesses or accidents. The definition of 'serious' was left to the parents, but these illnesses included three cases of epilepsy (two mild and said to be due to brain damage at birth and one very severe and requiring special school and later permanent hospitalisation), as well as six cases of depression (four of them during adolescence and all lasting a few weeks or months). In addition one child had a kidney removed, two had quite recently been diagnosed as diabetics, and several had suffered from illnesses such as meningitis, pneumonia, rheumatic fever, jaundice, glandular fever and osteomyelitis. Eleven adoptees had had accidents — not surprisingly all but one of them boys. Several fractures were sustained as a result of sports and games. One boy had been killed on his motorbike at the age of 17. His parents, nevertheless, were more than willing to talk of the happy years they had had with their son. Another young man lost an arm in a motorcycle accident and two were seriously but not permanently injured in car accidents.

Almost all the adoptive parents seemed to have coped very well with health problems as they occurred, and they made appropriate use of community medical facilities. There was no tendency except in a case of an actual genetic condition for parents to suggest that responsibility for medical problems or slight physical handicaps might lie with the children's heredity or with the fact of their adoption, nor in general was any apparent relationship found between these problems and the adjustment the children were making now as adults, or the satisfaction parents and children felt with each other.

Parents seemed much better able to cope with medical problems or slow mental development than with behaviour problems, at least to the extent of not letting ill-health or even serious backwardness alienate them from their children. However, the range of response and outlook found in the families is shown in two examples. A girl with very poor eyesight and 'inoperable strabismus' (combined with very slow mental development) had parents who resented her multiple handicap and saw the journeys to hospital and clinic throughout her childhood as an unpleasant chore which had been thrust upon them. By contrast the foster parents who took the baby with a heart condition adopted him when he was 2½ years old and at 5 years he had corrective heart surgery. In spite of some residual heart defect and little educational achievement this youngster was always very well accepted in this family of older adopters where the father had been married previously and already had grown-up children.

PROBLEMS OF DEVELOPMENT

Three families in the study (2 per cent) had a child who required special education because of mental subnormality, but only one of them (now said to have a mental age of 4 or 5 years) had to be permanently hospitalised. This child was placed at 3 months with a childless middle-class couple for direct adoption. His retarded development was noted early and the adopters sought opinions from several sources, which usually advised them to seek residential care for him. When they applied for and received a second child for adoption, they did not mention the first child's developmental problems; they felt the agency would think they were complaining. They did their best to care for this child at home, but when the mother's health began to break down they reluctantly placed him in residential care. He was then 7. He is said to be contented and visits home regularly every third weekend. His parents are, of course, disappointed, but there is no bitterness or blame and they believe it could have been the same if the child had been born to them. They felt he was their child right from the start and they still feel that way.

The other two children with subnormal development were placed as foster children when they were 6 months old. When one of these children was legally adopted at 2½ by middle-aged and hard-working foster parents who already had a grown-up son, the slow development had not been noticed. But when this little girl started school, she was unable to get along there and soon spent most of the day rocking. A day school for educationally subnormal children was recommended, but her condition deteriorated there and she was transferred to an ESN boarding school which soon diagnosed her as ineducable and sent her to a day training centre which at 24 she was still attending when we saw her. She is financially supported by social security since she is unemployable. Unfortunately, this young woman's subnormal development is complicated by behavioural symptoms which over the years have necessitated out-patient treatment, and more recently five months in a psychiatric ward. (She is one of the five cases of depression mentioned above.) She is difficult to live with, but the parents accept her and manage to get along with her most of the time. The adoptive mother, particularly, takes some satisfaction in having given a home to a child she feels would otherwise have been in residential care but she is disappointed that the girl is not more companionable, and both parents, now quite elderly, dread the idea that she will not be able to live outside an institution when they are gone.

The third educationally subnormal child, a boy, came from a background of subnormality and was fostered with a warm-hearted childless couple with extremely simple tastes and few expectations. They longed to adopt this child and he wanted nothing more than to be adopted so that his position in the family would be secure. These parents were not at all troubled by his slow development, but because of it the agency was opposed to adoption and did not consent until the boy was 11 years old. Still later the adopters finally had a child born to them, a girl, who also is retarded in development but well accepted and well loved. The son is now a coalman, as his adoptive father was in his youth; he had held his job for several years, likes his work and is self-supporting. This young man is still living at home where he is more than welcome in this close-knit family. He has friends of both sexes and appears to lead a normal life in the pattern of the young working man.

In addition to these three adoptees formally declared to be educationally subnormal and attending special schools, there were 26 (16 per cent) whose parents described them as slow to learn, although able to cope with ordinary education. As it was the parents' view we wanted, definition of the word 'slow' was left to them, and we found very different conceptions of slowness. There were four or five children who probably performed at only a marginally higher level than some of those attending special schools for the educationally subnormal. Though they remained in regular school until 15, they never acquired much knowledge of basic skills such as reading, writing and arithmetic. One boy was said to be unable to understand the business end of the family farm, and another could not write and figure well enough to cope with the family grocery. Both these boys were a disappointment to their parents in this regard but not rejected.

A quite different conception of slowness was found in two very intellectual families where the parents told us that the child's IQ was over 120, but that 'this was not high enough to do more than O levels', whereas a university education was expected as the normal course of events in their families and necessary to a good life. One said that they could tell from an early age that the child would not be academic, though they loved him nevertheless.

Various other children were described by their parents as 'not bright' though perhaps this says as much about the expectations of the parents as it does about the development of the children. At any rate all 26 so-called 'slow learners' are now employed and self-supporting except two girls, one married and financially dependent on her husband, and the other, mentioned earlier, who keeps house for her father.

Occasionally, accelerated development can be a problem too. A gifted child can be difficult to bring up and one family in the project encountered this problem. There was no reason to suppose this baby's development would be in any way exceptional when she was placed with hard-working, warm-hearted adopters with several other children. She was a very poor sleeper and developed into a very anxious, nervous little girl. Professional help was sought when she was 5 years old. After testing, the parents were told this child had an IQ of 170 and was a 'genius', who would be hard to bring up and might have to be taught outside the school system. Home teaching was tried for a while, but the child was so vulnerable to the slightest stress that the family were advised to try a boarding school for maladjusted children. She got on well there, but left without any qualifications and is now a cheerful, contented wife and mother with no indication of exceptional intellectual ability. Her parents think her intelligence is now average and they accept that 'because of her nerves she was not able to fulfil the promise she showed as a young child. It appears that much harm was done by the way the early tests were interpreted to the family, and the real difficulty appears to have been more a personality problem than a matter of giftedness.

PERSONALITY AND BEHAVIOUR PROBLEMS

Parents were asked what behaviour or personality problems the children had had over the years. Specific behaviour was not suggested; it was left to them to tell us what behaviour they remembered as problematic because we wanted to know what they had seen as difficult. Just over half, 54 per cent, said there had been problems at one time or another. Some of these were very serious and persisted even now, but others were very mild or temporary problems. (It is important to remember that, as the Isle of Wight study stressed, most normal children go through periods of stress or strain leading to phases of emotional upset and difficult behaviour.) Included among the problems mentioned by parents in the project were many which bring children to child guidance clinics and a very few that bring them to schools for maladjusted children or to correctional institutions. Girls and boys were about equally subject to problem behaviour but the kind of acting out which brought them into conflict with the law was largely confined to boys.

Early childhood difficulties included stammering and indistinct speech, temper tantrums, nightmares, fantasies and persistent enuresis. A number of children were so shy and insecure that parents had to put considerable effort into creating opportunities for them to make friends and enjoy social activities. But many more children were tense, overactive, aggressive or acting out, and this was usually at its worst in adolescence. One such boy, always overactive, drove himself so hard that he had a brief breakdown while at university. Others were aggressive or disrupting at school or truanted from school. Parents tended to find aggressive children more difficult to understand and sympathise with than those who were shy and withdrawn.

Some of the behaviour described would have been considered disquieting by most parents, but there was a little girl whose mother reported her as 'stealing' at 6 years of age when she took a small item from home to show at school without first getting permission, and another youngster whose mother spoke of him as a 'kleptomaniac' at age 5. There were a few parents, like these last, who were so concerned about a child's heredity (real or imagined) that they tended to draw sinister conclusions even from the most childish behaviour. Another adoptive mother spoke of her strong-willed daughter as being very like herself, but when referring to this trait in the girl she called it 'perversity' and indicated it had resulted in almost constant conflict during the adolescent years.

Late nights were an issue in a great many homes and many children who otherwise conformed to what was expected of them rebelled at parental restrictions on hours and dating, especially during late adolescence. Some of these adoptees, now grown up and building families of their own, volunteered during our interview with them that they had come to see the need for parents to set some limits.

There were several instances of sexual acting out among the girls in the study, but very few out-of-wedlock pregnancies were reported. Two girls had abortions to end pregnancies and one of these girls became pregnant again and this time relinquished her baby for adoption. This latter girl was extremely rebellious in adolescence, but with the help of her very understanding and tolerant family she came through this difficult period and has grown into a woman who is happily married and law-abiding, though she seems rather shallow emotionally.

Another girl with a very disturbed adolescence kept her illegitimate baby and later made what sounds to be a most unpromising marriage. A girl, mentioned earlier because of her poor adjustment, had an illegitimate child that she left mostly in the care of her rejecting adoptive mother, and another young woman with parents who were perhaps a little too easy-going had an illegitimate baby whom her adoptive mother apparently quite happily adopted.

Official statistics (Thompson and Peretz, eds. 1977, p. 11) show that in 1975 one in six legitimate births to women under 25 was conceived before marriage and that nearly a third of the women who married at ages under 20 in 1976 were pregnant on their wedding day. So it is not surprising that there were at least three young women in the study who married the fathers of their unborn children. All these marriages soon broke down and the girls were working hard to support the children.

That the families seem to have been reasonably tolerant of illegitimate pregnancies probably reflects the change in attitudes during the lifetime of these adoptees. There may also have been the half-expectation that the girls would follow in the footsteps of their unmarried mothers, as some of the parents viewed this kind of behaviour as hereditary. In fact two adopters said exactly that and another spoke of her daughter's sex appeal which she viewed as genetic, while still another said of her daughter: 'Of course, she is sexually attractive or she wouldn't be here, would she?' At the same time this mother expressed concern because she thought the girl's rather puritanical attitude to premarital sex was a bit old-fashioned.

Seven children (all boys) were said to have presented behaviour difficulties (uncomplicated by slow development or serious medical problems) from a very early age and which continued even into the present. In every instance these were cases where one or both parents had never accepted the reality of adoption. They either saw the child's fate as already sealed or else could not love a child they were not able to mould into a likeness of the one they might have had naturally. In these families trouble started early and gained momentum under increasing rejection. One father said 'All was well until the boy reached the age of 7 and began to have a mind of his own' and another described his son as 'Nothing but trouble since he was 3 years old'.

In the first case the boy was nervous and had many fears which he apparently handled in a different way when he got older, becoming restless, aggressive and overbearing, and as an adult ruthlessly competitive and irresponsible. The other boy had temper tantrums as a very young child, then began petty stealing followed by running away and sexual acting out in early adolescence, and more recently by a broken marriage, homelessness and drug pushing.

A third child was considered a problem from 18 months of age when he began head-banging and holding his breath after a second child was taken for adoption. Later, the natural child that the adopters had longed for was born to them and the first adopted child seemed even less desirable for he was then lying, stealing at home and in the neighbourhood and not achieving in school. This boy has now made a satisfactory life for himself apart from and quite different from his adoptive family's life-style.

Another of the problem children cried almost from the day he was placed as a foster child and he was said to be 'out of control' when scarcely more than a toddler. At 11 he began stealing, first from his very limited and rejecting mother (who then for the first time told him he was adopted), next from cars and then by housebreaking. At the request of his mother he was sent to an approved school where he adjusted very well. His mother gave her consent to an early marriage and afterwards said: 'Thank God for that, he is gone.' In spite of an unhappy childhood this boy is said to be surprisingly free of bitterness towards his parents and is thought by them to be a good husband and father.

Another boy was a head banger as a young child, stammered, was aggressive and had a 'fierce temper'. He was a bright child but temperamentally very different from the adoptive parents, who tried their best but were never able to understand him with the result that they were always in conflict. This boy started smoking at 12 and not long afterwards was on drugs and acting out aggressively in the community. Child guidance clinic followed by a boarding school placement had little effect, and after being involved with some other boys in an assault he was sent to borstal. He has not been in any further trouble but has not settled and seems always to be searching for something.

The other two boys whose families thought of them as long-term problems both lost their mothers early, one by death, the other by divorce. The first was brought up in a high delinquency area by an adoptive relative who gave him excessive freedom and had little interest in his school work or recreational activities, since she already had her hands full with her own family. He began stealing at an early age, joined an organised gang of boys with whom he got into more serious trouble, was placed on probation, then sent to borstal and finally to jail for taking part in a gang mugging.

The other boy is said to have been a 'wonderful baby but he changed overnight when he started school'. His mother placed extreme emphasis on cleanliness, but the boy was encopretic and also seemed to delight in getting as dirty as possible. His relationship with his mother was broken off when she left the home prior to a divorce. His father remarried and the step-mother tried hard to win the boy's confidence and be a mother to him, but he lied and stole from her and resented the children of her previous marriage. The father and step-mother recognised some of the boy's needs and at the suggestion of their GP consulted a child guidance clinic and attended for several weeks, but treatment ended when they found the psychiatrist's interpretation of the boy's behaviour so far-fetched that they concluded psychiatry was 'an utter waste of time'. This boy left home at the minimum school-leaving age and is no longer in touch with his family.

These depressing cases are given in detail not because there were many others like them but because they are examples of how problems can arise from a combination of several adverse factors, sometimes originating in a personality trait in the child but more often in factors in the environment.

Delinquency

Of the 160 sets of parents interviewed, 21 (13 per cent) said the adoptee had been known to the police at some time. Many of the offences were very minor; others were much more serious. They ranged from such things as trespassing on private property, shoplifting from Woolworth's at age 11, taking part in a political demonstration or riding a friend's motorbike under age and without a licence, on up through reckless driving and drug-taking, housebreaking, car theft and mugging.

Not all the cases known to the police came to court. Of those that did the outcome included several prison sentences ranging from one month to three years. Other adoptees spent periods in a remand home, approved school, detention centre or borstal. Only two instances of delinquency before the age of 10 were reported. It was in the age group 11 to 16 that anti-social behaviour most often showed up and those whose later offences resulted in imprisonment nearly all had been picked up for juvenile delinquency before they were 16.

There were eleven adoptees who had been seriously delinquent, and among them they had committed nine thefts (mostly cars), five drug offences and two acts of violence (mugging and attacking in a gang). Most of these people have been mentioned previously because their law-breaking followed a long series of other problems. In almost every one of these cases of anti-social behaviour, especially the more serious ones, it is possible now with hindsight to see what probably went wrong in these families. As with the problem behaviour described in the previous section, there was nearly always a number of different causes for the actions which brought this group of 21 adoptees into conflict with the law.

Factors related to emotional or behaviour problems

As we have seen, 86 or just over half of the adopted persons were considered by their parents to have shown one or more emotional or behaviour problems at some time while growing up, including the anti-social behaviour already mentioned which brought some into major or minor conflict with the law. Taking all these problems together, from enuresis or stammering to car theft and mugging, let us look at any relationship which was found to exist between these problems and the factors studied.

In contrast to research based on adopted children seen in child guidance clinics, no apparent relationship was found with the age of the child or the adopters at placement. Nor was any found with the number of previous living arrangements the child had had or his ordinal place in the adoptive family, nor with the adoptive mother's employment outside the home or with the adoptee's present attitude to his birth parents.

As regards social class the picture is different. A fair number of parents in all social classes had problems with their children (Table 11.1). However, the

Table 11.1 *Adoptees' behaviour problems, related to social class of adoptive father*

	Social class of adoptive father									
	Social class I		Social class II		Social class III		Social class IV		Total	
	no.	%	no.	%	no.	%	no.	%	no.	%
Behaviour problems										
No problems	13	52	18	42	38	48	5	38	74	46
Problems	12	48	25	58	41	52	8	62	86	54
Total	25	100	43	100	79	100	13	100	160	100

Table 11.2 *Adoptees in conflict with the law, related to social class of adoptive father*

	Social class of adoptive father									
	Social class I		Social class II		Social class III		Social class IV		Total	
	no.	%	no.	%	no.	%	no.	%	no.	%
Offences										
None	23	92	38	88	68	86	8	62	137	86
One or more	2	8	5	12	9	11	5	38	21	13
Not covered	—	—	—	—	2	3	—	—	2	1
Total	25	100	43	100	79	100	13	100	160	100

adopters in semi-skilled manual work (social class IV) somewhat more often had children with behaviour problems and their children were three times as likely to have been in some trouble with the police (Table 11.2). The current occupations of the young adults themselves also were rather closely related

Table 11.3 *Behaviour problems, related to adoptees' social class based on their own current employment*

	Social class of adoptees based on their own employment										
	Social classes I and II		Social class III		Social classes IV and V		Armed forces		Not employed (housewives, students, etc.)		Total	
	no.	%	no.	%	no.	%	no.	%	no.	%	no.	%
Behaviour problems												
No problems	26	54	26	46	2	12	5	83	15	45	74	46
Problems	22	46	30	54	15	88	1	17	18	55	86	54
Total	48	100	56	100	17	100	6	100	33	100	160	100

Table 11.4 *Adoptees' earlier behaviour problems, related to basis on which they had been received into their families*

	Basis on which adoptees were received into their families							
	Adoption only		Fostering with a view to adoption		Fostering only		Total	
	no.	%	no.	%	no.	%	no.	%
Behaviour problems								
No problems	37	48	34	49	3	21	74	46
Problems	40	52	35	51	11	79	86	54
Total	77	100	69	100	14	100	160	100

to the existence of problems (Table 11.3). No less than 15 of the 17 young people now in unskilled or semi-skilled employment were said to have had emotional or behaviour problems while growing up compared with about half of those in other classified occupations. Indeed only one of the ten who had been detained in some form of custody had ever been employed in anything except semi-skilled or unskilled manual work. The complex and controversial issues raised by any discussion of class have been the subject of many books and learned papers and are far beyond the scope of this study. All we can do here is to report the facts as we found them.

Problems were reported equally in children placed directly for adoption and in those adopted after fostering. However, when the 14 children who were taken *only* as foster children without a view to adoption were separated from the others, it was found that a much higher proportion of these children had had problems (11 of the 14) (Table 11.4).

It is also noteworthy that problems were reported in eight of the nine children in families who subsequently fostered an additional child. These foster children were of various ages, at least three of them older than the adopted child. They usually came at the request of an agency or of a family friend, and they stayed for varying periods of time. In one of the cases where the later foster child was the elder, the adoptive father said they had never adopted that child because the adoptive mother could not love him and the father felt this boy had led the adopted son in the study into 'a life of crime'. In another case a later foster child was returned to the agency after two years because of 'behaviour problems and background', and in another the adoptive mother had found the foster son more satisfactory than the adopted son.

It appears that trouble began early in some homes with the child having difficulties in settling, as 18 of the 21 children whose parents said they had been slow to settle, or had never really settled, had behaviour problems later on, compared with only half of those who had settled relatively soon after placement. Also, adoptees with parents who had criticisms or doubts about them early in the placement were more often the ones who acted out in the community and got into trouble with the police (one in three compared with one in ten). There seems to be some association, too, between delinquent behaviour and the extent of the father's involvement with the child over the years. Only one in ten was involved with the law when the adoptive father, as happened in most of the project families, was emotionally involved with the child in his upbringing, but of the thirteen whose fathers were not much involved or who were separated early by death or divorce, six had been in trouble.

As we might expect, parents who felt they had always had a close relationship with their child, even during adolescence and beyond, less often had a child with problems, and when they had been able to maintain an atmosphere of well-being and security in the home during all those years the children very much less often had behaviour problems than when there had been conflict, anxiety or insecurity in the home.

Doubts and anxieties about adoption itself showed up as related to the children's emotional and behaviour difficulties. The frequency with which adoption was discussed did not seem to matter much except that problems were reported in six of the seven families where the subject had been mentioned only once. However, as shown in Table 11.5 the discomfort

Table 11.5 *Adoptees' earlier behaviour problems, related to their discomfort in discussing adoption with parents*

	Discussion with parents							
	Comfortable		Uncomfortable		Not covered		Total	
	no.	%	no.	%	no.	%	no.	%
Behaviour problems								
No problems	26	59	18	33	1	33	45	45
Problems	18	41	36	67	2	67	56	55
Total	44	100	54	100	3	100	101	100

adoptees felt about raising the subject with their parents was closely associated with their behaviour. The delinquents had particular problems in this regard. We were able to interview only 12 of the 21 adoptees who were said to have run into trouble with the law, but of these only 4 were satisfied with the information they had been given about their adoption and background; 9 of the 12 did not feel comfortable in discussing these matters with their parents, and in fact 5 of them were so uncomfortable that they had never done so.

Feelings of being very different from their adoptive family, or not being treated as though they were a natural child of the family, were associated with behaviour problems. Three-quarters of those who felt no likeness to their parents had problems, compared with less than half who felt there were similarities, and virtually all had problems when they felt they had not been treated as a natural child of the family. The subtle but important questions of whether parents considered the adoptees as their 'own' children and whether in turn they were regarded as 'real' parents were relevant to behaviour as they were to so many of the issues considered in previous chapters. There were fewer children with problems when parents felt the child was their own, but as previously explained, we are inclined to think this is very much a two-way thing, that feeling like a real parent to the child results in commitment, better handling and fewer problems, but also that behaviour problems may tend to make some parents feel the child is not their own, particularly if they have built up an image of the more perfect child who might have been born to them.

Parents with a tendency to rely on heredity more often had children with behaviour problems, particularly children who acted out their problems in an anti-social way, but here, too, cause and effect are not clear enough for us to be able to say how many of them had always held this view and how many had acquired it as a convenient explanation for their child's unacceptable behaviour.

A few comments by parents will serve to illustrate the kind of thinking that often lay behind the confidence some parents showed in heredity as the source of their children's problems. One father believed his daughter's 'obsessive tidiness' and her 'hardness towards people' might be due to the possibility of her birth father being a German prisoner-of-war, as he believes Germans have these traits.

On the basis of a card received from her, one family assessed their son's birth mother and her family as illiterate. Equating illiteracy with dishonesty and delinquency and searching for a cause for the boy's delinquency, they wondered if his stealing from them and the neighbours, and his more recent drinking habits, were usual in his biological family and might have been accepted by that family as normal to their life-style. Another mother commented about her daughter: 'The first thing is heredity; it is much more significant than environment because it is always coming out, as in her touch of occasional vulgarity, for example, short mini-skirts in adolescence.'

And then there was the mother who was not at all surprised when the police called on her to say her teenage son had been caught stealing coins from telephone kiosks. She said she had been told by the agency that the boy's putative father was in prison. 'So what can you expect?' she said. 'It's in his bloodstream.'

Help with problems

When the adopters were asked if they would have liked more help from the placement agency, there was little enthusiasm for this idea. More than 20 years ago agencies were not very well qualified to help with problems of child-rearing, so perhaps it is not surprising that these adoptive parents did not see their agency as a source of assistance when problems arose with the child. Even those families where an agency social worker had visited for several years until the foster child was legally adopted did not see her as a source of help to them as parents, but rather as a friendly visitor who came periodically to check up on the child's progress and see that he was not being mistreated or neglected. In two or three instances where workers insisted upon children being told of their foster status, parents were critical of them for interfering as the children then had to be told at a time or in a way that foster parents felt was wrong.

The attitude of many direct adopters was that the agency was only an intermediary for getting the child and they could not imagine seeking its help in bringing up the child. This was exemplified by the mother whose response to the question was 'Good God! What would we do that for?' Others said that consulting the agency would have made them feel incapable as parents or as though the child were not theirs. One dissatisfied and unhappy mother said she would have been ashamed to go to her agency about such a problem; they would have wondered where she had gone wrong. Other parents felt the child was their responsibility and they wanted to go it alone. They said that if any help had been required it would have been available through the channels open to all parents, but few of them had actually used these resources. It is interesting that Rutter *et al.* (1970) in their Isle of Wight study also found that rather few parents in the community sought help from child guidance or other community counselling agencies.

Personality and behaviour problems affected family relationships much more seriously than even chronic illness or slow development needing special schooling. And not only did adopters find such problems harder to cope with themselves, they also found it more difficult to seek or obtain appropriate help.

Table 11.6   *Source of help with behaviour problems*

	no.	%
Family doctor only	9	11
Child guidance clinic only	13	15
Residential placement including court commitments	8	9
Handled by family alone	56	65
Total	86	100

Table 11.6 shows how adopters handled the behaviour and personality problems their children presented over the years. Behaviour which brought the young people into conflict with the law took the matter out of their parents' hands, but most of the 21 adoptees who were delinquent also had difficulties of other kinds and these have been included in the table.

Of the 86 children showing problems, only 8 had received any form of residential care, and this had lasted for periods of some six weeks to two or three years. Residential care usually had been preceded by out-patient treatment at a child guidance clinic. There also were 13 other cases where parents had sought advice at a child guidance clinic. Unfortunately, in most cases the adopters' experience with the clinic was not very satisfactory and these parents were critical. They felt the clinics had not been helpful, had not understood about adoption and had concentrated on diagnosis without doing much about treatment. When treatment was undertaken in a few cases, its aims were not understood, and when parents themselves were in treatment they felt the clinic staff must feel they were responsible for the child's problems, whereas they themselves felt it was the child who needed to be treated and his behaviour changed. Staff and parents seldom seemed to be on the same wave length and most parents withdrew in a short time feeling it was not worthwhile.

It may be that the adoptive parents were particularly reluctant to seek or accept professional advice because they already felt under scrutiny in the parental role, and also for some it meant opening up latent feelings of inadequacy because of infertility. However, the literature seems to indicate that, if anything, undue numbers of adopted children have been seen in child guidance clinics both in this country and in the United States (Humphrey and Ounsted, 1963; Sweeney *et al.*, 1963; Schecter *et al.*, 1964; Borgotta and Fanshel, 1965) and it is often suggested that adopters are quicker than most parents to seek such help. At any rate, in this study, two-thirds of the parents with children who had emotional or behaviour problems either did not consider the problems severe enough to need professional intervention or decided they could handle them within the family. Some of the problems were indeed minor or transitory and probably did not require professional help, but some which persisted or became serious might have responded to treatment at an early stage, if help had been readily available in some form acceptable to adoptive parents.

The whole question of follow-up services for adoptive families will be considered in more detail in the final chapter, but it may be useful to mention one or two points here. The largest number of parents who were able to see in the agency a source of possible help thought this might have been desirable many years after the adoption when problems had arisen, most often during the child's adolescence. They saw this as consisting of additional information from case files which would help to explain the child's difficult temperament, behaviour or school failure, and give them something on which to pin the cause of the difficulties. Two or three did wish they had had real help with a child who had problems they had not been able to understand or cope with, and one family actually had requested and received help from their agency in handling a problem that arose in adolescence.

Chapter 12

---◆---

EXPECTATION AND ACHIEVEMENT

In making the difficult decision to place their babies for adoption, the natural mothers of the adoptees in this study were hoping this would ensure a better chance in life than they themselves could provide. The agencies, too, were concerned to secure a good start for the children on whose behalf they were selecting substitute parents. For their part, adopters came forward to offer their home to a needy child in the confident expectation that they could provide opportunities as well as affection. It is therefore a useful of the 'success' of adoption placements to examine how the children responded to the opportunities offered them and whether they fulfilled their adoptive parents' educational and vocational expectations.

EDUCATION

As we have seen, parents felt that school had been the most frequent area of friction with their children, and when the adoptees themselves were asked about their school experience only half said they had enjoyed even one of the schools they had attended. The other half had merely tolerated school, had found it irrelevant or had thoroughly disliked it. As might be expected, those who later went to university were most often those who had liked school.

This attitude to school would lead one to expect poor results and early drop-out, but this was not in fact the case. Only 45 (27 per cent) of the 164 adopted people in the study had left school at 15. This compares very favourably with their contemporaries in the general population where the majority still left school at the minimum statutory age (Thompson and Peretz, eds, 1977, p. 12). Furthermore, one in three (56) of the adoptees took some form of advanced education beyond the O level or ordinary school certificate (Table 12.1). Of these 56, 7 ended their formal education with A levels or a higher school certificate, but the remaining 49 went on to university, technical college, hospital or teachers' training college where 20 earned degree-level qualifications and the others a diploma, certificate or SRN qualification. Three now have higher degrees, one a PhD. Science, including engineering, was the most popular degree just as it is among UK students generally (Thompson and Peretz, eds, 1977, p.14), but law, medicine, maths, English, music and others were represented. Teacher training was the most common course of study for a diploma, but others had studied such subjects as accounting, architecture, art and design, nursing,

Table 12.1 *Educational achievement of adoptees*

	no.	%
University	17 ⎫	10 ⎫
Non-university degree, diploma or certificate	32 ⎬ 56	20 ⎬ 34
A levels or higher school certificate	7 ⎭	4 ⎭
O levels or ordinary school certificate	42	26
Vocational training or apprenticeship requiring no academic qualifications	19	12
No educational qualifications either academic or vocational	45	27
Not covered	2	1
Total	164	100

hotel management, librarianship. With 20 (12 per cent) of our 22-to 27-year olds earning a degree-level qualification, these young people compare favourably with other young people in the United Kingdom aged 25 among whom 7 per cent (1 in 14) are said to have such a qualification (Thompson and Peretz, eds, 1977, p.10).

Another 12 per cent (19 adoptees) had completed apprenticeships or taken other vocational training, either full- or part-time, which did not require academic qualifications but nevertheless fitted them for skilled employment. It seemed that being qualified for a job, even a relatively simple one, represented a very worthwhile achievement and was closely linked with these young people's self-image and satisfaction. Every one of those with a university qualification whom we were able to interview, said he or she was pleased with the way life was going at this time. In fact, those who had taken other advanced education or job qualification were also much more inclined to be satisfied with their current life-style than those without it.

It is well known that education is closely related to social class, that children from privileged homes tend to stay in school longer and much more often take advanced education (Bamford), 1977; Thompson and Peretz, eds, 1977, pp.10,74). The adopted people in the study were no exception, for more than half of those with adoptive fathers in social class I or II occupations had been educated beyond O level, but only one in five of those with parents in other occupations had that much education. Attaining O levels alone did not seem to be associated with social class, but at the bottom rung of the attainment ladder class showed up again. More than one in three of the adoptees in families in social classes III and IV had no qualifications of any kind compared with one in five in social class II. Of the 26 young people with adoptive fathers in professional and managerial occupations there was only one who was without some qualification. The overall good educational achievement of the adoptees appears to be related to the fact that so many were in professional, semi-professional or managerial families and relatively few were in families where the father was in semi-skilled manual work (Table 12.2).

Table 12.2 *Adoptees' educational achievement, related to social class of adoptive father*

	Social class of adoptive father											
	Social class I		Social class II		Social class III		Social class IV		Social class V		Total	
	no.	%	no.	%	no.	%	no.	%	no.	%	no.	%
Education												
Advanced education (university, non-university degree or diploma, A levels)	14	*54*	23	*52*	16	*20*	3	*23*	—	—	56	*34*
O levels or ordinary school certificate	8	*31*	9	*20*	21	*26*	3	*23*	1	*100*	42	*26*
Vocational training or apprenticeship (no academic qualifications	3	*11*	3	*7*	11	*14*	2	*15*	—	—	19	*12*
No educational qualifications either academic or vocational	1	*4*	9	*21*	30	*37*	5	*39*	—	—	45	*27*
Not covered	—	—	—	—	2	*3*	—	—	—	—	2	*1*
Total	26	*100*	44	*100*	80	*100*	13	*100*	1	*100*	164	*100*

A great deal of research in adoption has been concerned with the relative influence of environment and heredity, since it is in adopted children that these factors can most easily be examined. Our study does not shed much additional light on the subject though it reinforces the general finding that both heredity and environment influence children's achievement. The information in case records was often inadequate for proper comparison of the child's biological and adoptive family. Their birth mothers were often young and the pregnancy sometimes interrupted their education or led to a change in employment, so the occupations listed on the case papers were not necessarily their regular work. Their father's occupation would have been a much more reliable indicator of family background, but this was not always recorded. In most instances little information was available about putative fathers, and what there was sometimes seemed of doubtful accuracy.

For all these reasons, comparison of the adoptees' biological and adoptive background is complicated and not very satisfactory. It is quite clear that in general the children moved up the social ladder at placement, but at the same time the agencies evidently were operating a process of rough matching, at least to the extent that children whose birth parents came from higher social classes tended to go to adoptive families of similar background. An examination of the adoptees' educational attainment and the class of their biological and adoptive parents shows that of the 56 with advanced educational attainment 24 (44 per cent) were known to have had one or both birth parents, or a maternal grandfather, employed in social class I or II occupations, but all except 4 of these also had an adoptive father in these occupations. Among them was one case in which the maternal grandfather, the putative father, the adoptive father and the adopted son were all in the same highly regarded profession.

It is obvious, too, that various factors were operating in the environment, among them the advantaged life-style of many of the adoptive families, the attention given to schooling including careful choice of schools, high expectations and a good deal of encouragement. For instance a young man who graduated very creditably from university was encouraged by his intellectual adoptive parents, although they knew that his birth parents and his maternal grandfather had little education as both had been employed in unskilled or semi-skilled work.

A man with no known musical ability in either his natural or adoptive family had gained a good musical education and was making music his life. In this case the adoptive family, although unacademic and not musical themselves, saw that the boy had talent and encouraged him to develop it. There were two young men with a university education where the motivation seems to have come entirely from within themselves, where nothing in their background or in the socioeconomic level of the adoptive homes would lead one to expect much intellectual interest or encouragement. One of these boys in particular worked very hard for an education. He convinced his parents, who were not themselves well educated, that he must go to university, and he worked weekends and holidays so that his staying on at school to prepare for university admission would not make life harder for them. He did well at university and is now a qualififed engineer, and the family is understandably proud of him.

In our opinion these findings indicate that both the child and adoptive parents, as well as the school, contributed to educational success or failure.

There was always what the child brought with him by way of natural ability and ambition, as well as all his parents put into it by providing security and encouraging him to develop his fullest potential, whatever that proved to be. In two or three cases parents reported an additional problem – that the school had expected failure or troublesome behaviour, or both, from fostered or adopted children.

EMPLOYMENT

On the day we interviewed their parents nine out of every ten of the adopted persons were either said to be self-supporting or were wives financially dependent upon their husbands. Most of the remainder were dependent upon student grants or were receiving appropriate social security benefits, but two were in hospital and one was in prison. Only two were dependent upon their parents, and one of these was the girl, mentioned several times earlier, who was earning her way as housekeeper for her father. The other was a poorly adjusted young man who was employed but nevertheless was not supporting himself or his estranged wife and children, and had returned home to live with his adoptive parents.

The interviews were carried out during a period of deepening financial recession, and a few had not found exactly the work they wanted, but unemployment had not been a problem. One young man with emotional problems had been made redundant but had subsequently decided to take further training. Of those usually gainfully employed, 85 per cent were thought by their parents to be happy in their work and in most cases their employment was appropriate to their training and experience.

Table 12.3   *Classification of adoptees' own current employment*

	no.	%
Social class I	14	9 ⎫ 30
Social class II	34	21 ⎭
Social class III	56	35
Social class IV	10	6 ⎫ 10
Social class V	7	4 ⎭
Not in classified employment	39	25
6 in armed forces		
22 housewives (1 housekeeper for father)		
4 students		
1 temporarily unemployed		
4 unemployable (ESN, epileptic, gaol)		
2 whereabouts and employment unknown to		
parents		
Total	160	*100*

Not surprisingly, some of those who had left school with no academic qualifications, and had taken no vocational training, were less satisfied in such unskilled jobs as they could get and they changed employment often. However, it could not be said that the adoptees on the whole were young people who showed a great deal of job mobility, as more than a third of those in employment had been with the same employer for three years or more and another third for at least a year. Some of those who had been in the same employment for less than a year were among the youngest in the study or had just completed their education and had been working only a short time on their first job. Table 12.3 shows the socioeconomic condition of the 121 adoptees who were employed at the time their parents were interviewed and also shows the whereabouts of the remaining 39 who were not in classified employment.*

PARENTAL ASPIRATIONS

It would be interesting to know how many children in the general population fulfil the ambitions their parents have for them. It is only natural that people should want the best for their children and many see education as the gateway to the good life. Parents often live their early lives over again through their children and count on them to achieve more than they themselves have done. Probably most parents begin by hoping a child will do well. They may dream of his attaining the rewards of higher education, but many are gradually forced to a more realistic view by the child's own limited ambitions or lack of scholastic aptitude.

For adoptive parents it may be particularly important for their children to be seen to be bright and ambitious, and never compared unfavourably with the children of relatives, neighbours or friends. This is part of the need adopters so often feel to convince themselves, when they are not too sure about it, that adoption is as good a way of parenthood as any other. If they see adoption as a handicap they may see education as a way to overcome this. Others may feel an achiever will help to compensate for the natural child they could not have. It may be inevitable that the hopes of adoptive parents are almost always high and sometimes quite unrealistic.

The findings of this study certainly confirm that adopters are ambitious for their children. Table 12.4 shows that nearly 40 per cent of those interviewed said the child had fallen short of their expectations. When these figures are compared with those for the adoptive parents' view of the overall adoption experience (see Table 5.1), it is quite evident that many who in general were well satisfied nevertheless said they were disappointed in the child's achievement. Whereas 85 per cent were satisfied overall, only 39 per

*The figures on this subject in Chapter 7 are limited to the 105 adoptees who could be interviewed, whereas reference here is to the 160 whose parents gave information about them.

cent felt that the adoptee had fulfilled or exceeded their expectations, though another 18 per cent had not set their sights on any particular level of attainment so could be content with whatever the child was able to achieve.

Table 12.4   *Adoptees' fulfilment of adoptive parents' expectations of achievement*

	no.	%
Fulfilled or exceeded expectations	62	39⎫ 57
No special expectations	29	18⎭
Fell short of expectations	63	39
Incompatible responses	4	3
Not covered	2	1
Total	160	100

Parents might be satisfied with a wide range of attainment. A former foster mother, mentioned in previous chapters in relation to her acceptance of her child's health and developmental problems, was quite proud of the fact that, though the boy had made very slow progress in school and had only an unskilled job, he was interested in getting ahead and was now taking evening classes in reading, writing and spelling.

Another boy who was in the slow stream all through school was a splendid athlete who competed for his school in national and international competitions. His family did not let his lack of academic achievement bother them, but encouraged his interest in sport and were very proud of him. He now has semi-skilled and satisfying employment, a family of his own and is a well-adjusted, likeable young man. This situation contrasts with another in which a girl, said to have an IQ of at least 115, showed up very poorly in school. Her parents believed she knew the subject matter but would not work in school. The parents did not like the way this child's personality was developing, and it seems likely that the resulting conflict with her parents may have had more to do with her school failure than poor intellectual development.

Different again were the families who remained disappointed with attainments which would have thrilled others. In one such family, the father was so disappointed that his son was not interested in sports or good at them that he was unable to think of him as anything but 'the office boy', although the son was, in fact, working in a highly skilled profession. One or two other families were distressed because the adoptee had left university with an ordinary degree rather than with honours.

When it came to employment, it could be said that parental hopes and expectations were again unrealistic in many instances, though perhaps if this same characteristic could be looked at in a sample of non-adopted families, the same situation would be revealed.

All the parents of adoptees now in professional or managerial work felt their ambitions had been accomplished (except that one of these families had no special expectations), whereas none of the 17 parents with a son or daughter in semi-skilled or unskilled work felt their goals for the child had been reached. Even those who were themselves only semi-skilled had wanted something better for their children and were often disappointed when this was not achieved (Table 12.5).

Table 12.5 *Adoptees' fulfilment of adoptive parents' expectations related to classification of adoptees' own employment*

	Classification of adoptees' own employment											
	Social class I		*Social class II*		*Social class III*		*Social class IV*		*Social class V*		*Total*	
	no.	*%*	*no.*	*%*	*no.*	*%*	*no.*	*%*	*no.*	*%*	*no.*	*%*
Fulfilment of expectations												
Fulfilled or exceeded expectations	13	93	18	53	16	28	—	—	—	—	47	39
No special expectations	1	7	6	18	11	20	3	30	1	14	22	18
Fell short of expectations	—	—	10	29	26	46	7	70	5	72	48	39
Incompatible responses	—	—	—	—	1	2	—	—	1	14	2	2
Not covered	—	—	—	—	2	4	—	—	—	—	2	2
Total	14	100	34	100	56	100	10	100	7	100	121*	100

* 121 in classified employment.

Fulfilment of the parents' expectations tied in with the extent to which they identified with the adopted child. Only 54 per cent of those who were disappointed in the child's achievement spoke of feeling the child to be their own, whereas 77 per cent of those who expressed satisfaction and 86 per cent who had formed no special expectations felt themselves identified with the child. It is, of course, difficult to disentangle cause and effect here.

When the adoptees who were interviewed were asked for *their* view of their parents' expectations, half said they had been high, and most of the others believed their parents had been moderately interested but without any special objectives for them. There were just three who thought their parents were uninterested in their school progress and four others who felt their parents had discouraged them by anticipating failure. Those who thought the expectations had been high were divided between those who thought their parents had put pressure on them to reach predetermined goals and those who had been allowed to progress at their own pace while their parents maintained their high expectations and encouraged them to do their best.

Adoptees with fathers in social class I or II occupations tended to believe their parents had had high expectations for them, but many parents in social classes III or IV were described as having been only moderately interested in their children's education and without special goals for them.

We have already seen that doing well at school and being employed now in satisfying work were linked with good adjustment, self-esteem and satisfaction with life, so it seems important to try to determine whether high parental expectation and pressure to achieve helped or hindered. The picture is not entirely clear, but it seems that the children achieved best when their parents held to high standards while letting them move ahead at their own rate. Over half (54 per cent) of those who took advanced education said their parents had done this, but only a relatively small proportion (16 per cent) of the others thought their parents had encouraged them without pushing and much more often thought their parents' interest in their education had been only moderate (Table 12.6).

Table 12.6 *Adoptees' view of parental expectations, related to educational achievement*

	Educational achievement					
	Education beyond O level		Education to O level or less		Total	
	no.	%	no.	%	no.	%
Adoptees' view of expectations						
High at own pace	20	54	11	16	31	30
High and pushed	6	16	14	21	20	19
Moderate interest	11	30	35	52	46	44
Uninterested	—	—	3	5	3	3
Expected failure	—	—	4	6	4	4
Total	37	100	67	100	104*	100

* Figures exclude one who could not be questioned on the subject.

It is also noteworthy that rather more of the adoptees who felt they had been pushed were said to have had personality or behaviour problems while growing up. Two in three of those experiencing parental pressure had these difficulties compared with only one in two of the adoptees whose parents' goals for them were more modest or where they were allowed to develop at their own pace even though expectations for them were high.

The whole question of reaching parents' goals was linked with whether or not the adopted person was thought to have made good use of the educational opportunities they had offered him. Indeed, this may have been the nub of the matter as far as parents' feelings were concerned. Most adopters feel they are offering something good and they want the gratification of seeing the child make effective use of it.

Just under half the parents thought their son or daughter had made good use of the opportunities offered for education or job training, no apparent difference being found between boys and girls in this respect. Another third of the parents said their child had made fair use of opportunities but they were sure he could have done better. Twenty-two families (14 per cent) believed the child had thrown away his chances, but four others chose to take the responsibility on themselves, saying they had not been able to offer very much.

Attitudes towards heredity showed up again here. Those who placed their faith in heredity much more often said the adoptees had rejected the chances they had given them, while those who believed in environment as more important were more inclined to think their children had availed themselves of what had been offered. Was this yet another example of a tendency to make a kind of scapegoat of heredity whenever things went wrong? Be that as it may, the use of opportunities was found associated with parents' present relationship with the adult son or daughter. When they thought the child had made good use of the chance he had had to develop his potential, more than three-quarters of the adopters felt the present relationship was close and satisfying. Only two-fifths felt that way when they believed the child could have done better, and very few parents now felt close to a child who in their opinion had wasted his opportunity.

.

PART FOUR

---◆---

FINDINGS AND IMPLICATIONS

Chapter 13

———◆———

FINDINGS AND THEIR IMPLICATIONS FOR PRACTICE

Readers will recall that, when this study was being planned, the intention was that its core should be a comparison of the outcome of two methods of adoption, namely, direct adoption placement and adoption by foster parents. However, as we have seen, the foster parent adopters were found to fall into two fairly distinct groups. There were the 'true' foster parents, who took the child expecting that he would quite likely be restored to his natural mother, and there were those who – in their own minds at least – were fostering with a view to adoption. Thus, in effect there were three groups to be considered, but the number of 'true' foster placements was so small – only 14 – that the experiences of these families cannot be conclusive. For most comparisons it has been necessary to combine all the foster parent adoptions even though a high proportion of these saw themselves as adoptive parents right from the start. This has inevitably complicated the analysis of findings and makes extra caution necessary in commenting on the basis for placement in relation to various measures of outcome. Even though the data did not permit us to distinguish between direct and foster parent adoptions as helpfully as we would have wished, we still feel the question was worth raising.

Fortunately, this disadvantage is reduced by the effect of the passage of time on the project families. We are concerned here with experiences which stretch back over more than 20 years. As time went on, the basis on which a child had joined his family became less important than their current life together. In regard to some of the most interesting and important aspects of adoptive family life, the question of whether or not the child had first been fostered was not particularly relevant, although it was always examined as a potential source of difference.

Another point which needs to be borne in mind when considering the study's overall findings is the interrelationship of a number of factors. For purposes of analysis and comparison one has to lift each aspect out of context for examination, but in reality there is a constant interweaving of influences. Association of factors is not necessarily cause and effect and in a descriptive study of this kind it has often been impossible to disentangle these extremely involved relationships. The relative importance of agency practice, adoptive parent responses and the child's reactions to these could not be determined at all exactly in this project and probably never will be because of the enormous variety of individual situations. All that can be done is to look at general trends and tendencies. In many instances these do indeed prove useful and interesting.

THE FINDINGS

By way of summarising the main findings, let us look again at the questions which the staff had in mind when the project started and see what answers finally were obtained.

Is adopting one's foster child more or less satisfying and rewarding than adopting a child directly from an adoption agency?

Little difference was found in the ultimate satisfaction of direct adopters and foster parent adopters. Looking back over the whole experience the vast majority in both groups assessed it as having been satisfying and rewarding in many ways and few of them regretted having embarked on it. However, a somewhat smaller proportion of the little group of 'true' foster parents were *very* satisfied with the overall experience, and of the eight very dissatisfied adopters six had fostered first. It also was noted that fewer of the 'true' foster parents had committed themselves to the child to the extent of regarding him as their own.

Thus, over the years the foster parent adopters enjoyed being parents but many looked back on the anxieties of the early years with strong feeling. Their problems were not so often with the child as with the agency or his birth mother. The latter had the power to give or withhold the child and the tremendous anxiety that she would not agree to their adopting him coloured the experience of most foster parents. Direct adopters worried about this too, but generally with less basis and for a much shorter period.

One of the most striking findings of the whole project was that virtually none of the adopters – no matter what route they had taken – saw any advantage in fostering first, and they saw a great many disadvantages. Of course foster parents who had not wanted to go on to adopt would not be included in this study. Nevertheless, one might expect that more than 10 of the 83 foster parent adopters would have found it a positive advantage to be able to get to know the child very well and see how things were going for an extended period before making the final commitment to adoption. It is clear, however, that the uncertainty of the fostering period created anxieties which outweighed any such benefits.

Does entering the family first as a foster child affect the long-term satisfaction or adult adjustment of the adoptee?

There was virtually no difference in the satisfaction with the adoptive experience expressed by the two groups of young adults. Four out of five of them were satisfied or very satisfied. Their adjustment, as assessed in the study, did show differences but only of degree. Overall, out of the 105 adoptees who were interviewed 31 per cent were rated A (excellent), 39 per cent B (good), 25 per cent C (marginal) and 5 per cent D (poorly adjusted). There was a tendency for those who had been fostered first to get a B rather than an A rating and of the six poorly adjusted young people in group D, five had been foster children.

Several of the former foster children remembered being worried about their situation in the family and having a different name. One cannot help wondering whether these worries played a part in causing the behaviour problems that were notable in the children originally taken only for fostering. No less than 11 of these 14 children were said to have shown difficult behaviour while growing up. Or were the 'true' foster children affected by the less-than-total commitment of their new parents referred to above? There seemed some tendency for the 'true' foster children to be undecided about who should be considered their real parents, but the numbers involved are too small for this interpretation to be more than very tentative. Research currently being carried out by Holbrook at the Institute of Psychiatry, University of London, may shed much more light on this point.

When there are long delays in legalising the adoption, does this affect the overall satisfaction of adopters or the satisfaction and adult adjustment of adoptees?

Neither overall satisfaction nor outcome was significantly affected by delays in achieving final adoption but, as already pointed out, adoptive parents and sometimes adoptees, too, had vivid and painful memories of their anxieties over uncertainty and postponements.

If the adoptive experience is satisfying to the parents, is it likely to be satisfying to the adoptee as well?

Although both parents and children were being asked in the interviews to comment on their whole experience of life together, inevitably they looked at this from different perspectives as well as over a different time-span. Whereas the adopters recalled their early years as parents, their feelings about the placement and their experience of seeing the child develop over the years, the young people could not remember their very early years and more often based their assessment on their experience as adolescents and young adults.

One would expect to find a high degree of congruence between satisfaction of adopters and adoptees. This was the case, but nevertheless one in five families differed in their assessment with some adoptees seemingly unaware of their parents' disappointment in them, and others unhappy about their adoption even though the parents expressed pleasure with the way things had gone.

A rather unexpected finding was that parental expectations were not merely high; quite often they could only be considered unreasonable. Many pushed their children hard to achieve in school, and good marks and exam results were very important in many families. The adoptees had rather mixed feelings about this. They clearly resented being pushed and liked it best when parents let them move ahead at their own pace. But they liked parents to hold to their high expectations, and when they had obtained higher education and the good jobs that resulted from this, they were well satisfied with themselves and with the adoption experience that had launched them on life so successfully. In other families, where little was expected, often little was achieved, and adoptees were then not very pleased with their humdrum jobs and the way their lives were going.

What was quite clear from the responses of both parents and young people was that an adoption did not have to be perfect to be seen as satisfying to those involved. All sorts of problems, conflicts and disappointments could occur and yet the overall feeling be very positive. As we have seen, the young people were much more likely to take the blame themselves for any problems. Their parents tended to blame heredity when things went wrong.

What is the effect on the adoptive family of contact between birth parents and adoptive parents?

A general answer could not be found to this question. Contact between the two sets of parents did not seem to be good or bad in itself. It meant different things to different people. Meeting the natural mother sometimes helped adopters to feel thoroughly entitled to the child, but it could work the other way and make a sense of entitlement almost impossible to achieve.

The adoptees seldom knew about these meetings. It was one of the many pieces of information which parents frequently withheld even when, in our view, it would have been likely to be beneficial to the children to be told. The children's satisfaction and adjustment were not directly linked with whether or not there had been contact, but no doubt they were affected indirectly by the influence of such meetings on their adoptive parents. Any feeling that adopters disapproved of their birth parents and background had a negative effect on adopted children. The former foster children more often knew how their adoptive parents felt about their birth mother and nearly a quarter of them thought these feelings were critical or disapproving. There were only a few instances of contact after the adoption had been legalised; a few adopters were agreeable to this and it was not necessarily harmful.

Are adopters and adoptees who perceive themselves as alike in some respects more often satisfied with their experience than those who see no such similarities?

This issue proved to be more interesting and relevant than expected. It had quite clearly been important to both parents and children that there were *some* points of likeness between them. To look alike, or share an interest, or have a similar personality or temperament all increased satisfaction and these points were often mentioned with pleasure. The question of cause and effect must remain open, so it would be misleading to say that similarities 'caused' successful placement, but they definitely were associated with it and often seem to have smoothed the path. Feelings were much more important than facts in this regard. Likenesses were perceived on very slender evidence. As with beauty, they were mainly in the eye of the beholder. If a child had emotional or behaviour problems, or achieved poorly, parents seldom saw him as like themselves or their relatives and he became more of an outsider, thus, one suspects, increasing the difficulties. If his achievement and adjustment were good, parents tended to identify readily with him, thus cementing the bonds.

Is the method and timing of the revelation of the child's adoptive status an important factor in his adult adjustment?

The study findings reinforce the importance of starting the explanations early, not because the timing in itself proved crucial, but because if delayed until after school entry the 'telling' was likely to be badly done and traumatic. That adoptees wish to learn of these things from their parents and not from outsiders was very evident.

Frequency of discussion proved much less important than a feeling of openness on the subject so that the child was able to ask questions. In general, however, parents found it difficult to offer information, and children, sensing their reluctance, found it hard and sometimes quite impossible to raise the subject.

Problems of communication proved disturbingly usual in the project families, though the adoptees often managed to be satisfied with remarkably little information about their origins. Contentment with the information given was linked with adoptee satisfaction, but contentment depended less on the quantity of data than on the child's feeling that his adoptive parents were not critical of his background.

Very striking indeed was the sense of insecurity in adoptive parents when it came to talking about background and birth parents. Even when things had gone well, and they had a close relationship with the young adult they had brought up from infancy, they still feared the power of the birth mother to wean him away and felt they might lose his affection. They 'told' the child because they realised they must, but they too often failed to explain adoption in ways that made any sense to the young child growing up and they failed to pass on background information which would have helped to increase the child's good self-image. Often they 'forgot' or distorted the information given them by their agency, even when the agency had taken the precaution of giving them this in writing, and it was evident that social workers have greatly underestimated the difficulty adopters have in explaining the facts to their children.

Are adopted people wanting to meet their birth parents usually those who are not satisfied with their experience in the adoptive family or not well adjusted as adults?
Other researchers such as Triseliotis (1974), and recent experience with adoptee access to birth records following the Children Act, 1975, have shown that there is a big difference between wanting more information about background and wanting to meet natural parents and establish a relationship with them.

This study confirmed this difference and also confirmed that a desire to make contact with birth parents is related both to adoptee satisfaction and to adjustment. Many of the adoptees interviewed in the project said they would welcome a little more information about themselves, but only 21 had been wishing to meet their first parents (perhaps just once), and of those there were 14 who were considered to be in the less well-adjusted C and D categories. Two, whose adopters knew their birth mothers, had already made contact, but did not plan to continue it. There were just two others who very much wanted to meet their birth parents and these really yearned for an on-going relationship with them, although one was frightened that the reality might be less rewarding than the fantasy.

Are parents likely to blame heredity when an adopted child shows problems while growing up?
Heredity proved more of a worry than it needed to be. Although adopters did not blame heredity for the problems of health or development which occurred while their children were growing up, they found behaviour and personality problems much more difficult to cope with, and there was a tendency for these behaviour problems to be linked with the parents' belief in the strong influence of heredity. Those parents who relied more on nature than on nurture also found it difficult to look upon an adopted child as their own, and both they and the children were less often satisfied with the adoption. To be satisfied, adoptive parents needed to feel that they were in themselves worthwhile people with much to give to a child and that they were fully entitled to bring up their adopted child.

Have things which social workers have traditionally considered important proved to be so?
This omnibus question was not set out as one to be answered as such, but it underlay the whole construction of the study and now provides a convenient way of summarising points not covered in the main questions.

Facts about the child
(a) Contrary to general belief (based largely on experience of adopted

children seen in child guidance clinics), neither age at placement, the number of previous moves nor having been in a residential nursery had any noticeable effect on the long-term outcome. Of course it is important to remember that all the children in the study were very young compared with many of the children now being placed for adoption.

(b) Boys grew up slightly less satisfied and less well adjusted than girls though the difference is too small to be significant in statistical terms.

(c) Physical handicaps and even very slow or limited mental development were not necessarily a bar to full acceptance by some adoptive parents.

Facts about the adopters

(a) The importance of *both* adopters truly accepting the adoptive relationship was demonstrated in the project. The effort of either parent to force a child into the likeness of one who might have been born to the family was markedly unsuccessful and resulted in much unhappiness.

(b) Adoptees were less satisfied when they had parents who seemed to them elderly, but they grew up just as well adjusted as those whose adopters were younger.

(c) Employment of the mother outside the home, though relatively unusual in the project families, did not affect satisfaction or adjustment.

(d) Social class of the adoptive father was associated with many other factors and its influence is therefore difficult to assess. As far as the adoptees' satisfaction goes, those in class I were both the most often satisfied and the best adjusted. Class III came next followed by II, and the rather small number of children placed in families where the adoptive father's occupation was social class IV were least often satisfied and well adjusted.

(e) Although there were instances where the ill-health of a parent caused a child much unhappiness, ill-health of fathers or siblings did not have long-term effects on adoptee adjustment. The mother's health was somewhat more important but much depended on the age of the child and severity and length of illness. But when either adoptive parent died, the child suffered far more grief and sense of loss than the remaining parent realises even now, and certainly nothing in the study would justify social workers paying any less attention than at present to the health of both adoptive applicants.

The emotional climate in the home

(a) The importance adoption workers have paid in recent years to the quality of personal relationships in the family is fully vindicated by the findings of this study. Plenty of affection, a cheerful and harmonious atmosphere, being allowed reasonable independence at an appropriate age and the absence of tension were all associated with a feeling of closeness in the

family and with satisfaction and good adjustment.
(b) The adopted child's ordinal place in the family did not matter and the presence or absence of siblings was not related to outcome. What was very important to all the adoptees was being treated as a full member of the family, i.e. like an 'own' child, and that parental attitudes were balanced so that the child was neither overwhelmingly the centre of attention nor pushed aside and ignored. Ten adoptees felt they had been treated as a step-child or foster child and only one of these was now making a good adjustment to adult life.

IMPLICATIONS FOR PRACTICE

Any research study about adoption outcome is likely to be full of implications for practice. These may be for change because past theories or methods are shown to have fallen short or the study may support the efficacy of past practice and thus help to ensure its continuation. It would be tedious to go over all the findings summarised in the first part of this chapter and examine the practice implications of each. Most of them are fairly obvious and seem to reinforce the findings of other studies and what experienced adoption workers have known for a long time. Affection, commitment, optimism and belief in the efficacy of happy family life are what count most. The crucial importance of detailed, careful and honest exploration of both adoptive applicants' attitudes, motives and expectations are pointed up over and over again in the situations analysed and described here. But there are three findings which seem so important to the current adoption scene that they need fuller consideration and discussion. *First* is the issue around which this study was planned and which is if anything even more crucial today when adoption is seen as the goal for so many older children separated from their families of origin. Is fostering with a view to adoption the best way of achieving that goal? *Secondly* comes the question of selecting a substitute family for a parentless child. Is there any validity in the old concept of 'matching'? *And finally*, what does the study tell us about services to the adoptive family? How and when can help be most effective?

Fostering with a view to adoption

The Thomas Coram Foundation children were never officially placed for adoption because at that time the Foundation was not an adoption agency. The purpose of the foster placement was to provide good family care for as long as necessary while the natural mother had a chance to consider the options carefully. She could make plans for the child to return to her, agree to adoption if the foster parents requested this, or she could leave the child to grow up in foster care. For children in the Foundation's care at this period adoption could only be achieved via fostering, both as a matter of agency policy and because almost none of the mothers would have given consent to adoption at the time the child was admitted. (If they had decided on adoption at this early stage they probably would have found their way to an adoption agency.)

These two factors, agency policy and difficulty over obtaining parental consents, are still the reasons for many children being placed in long-term foster homes by numerous voluntary and statutory child care agencies. In today's different social work scene the same constraints and anxieties still operate. In fact most of the children now being placed in substitute families have some complicating factor of family situation, age, health or behaviour which, on the face of it at least, might make direct adoption seem risky or impossible.

Until the Children Act, 1975, is fully implemented and the new 'freeing' procedures make it possible for an agency to obtain a court ruling on whether a child can be considered 'free' for adoption, there will continue to be many instances where the agency plan is to work towards adoption even though the consent of the natural parents is unobtainable and grounds for dispensing with it are not watertight. In these situations the only course open may be to seek long-term foster parents willing to accept an ambiguous relationship. In other cases, however, the natural parents' consent would be forthcoming quite readily, but the agency holds back preferring what seems to be the safe route of a fostering placement which may – or may not – develop gradually into adoption. Indeed in many agencies children beyond infancy are *always* fostered first.

This study's finding that the children adopted by foster parents were ultimately just as often well adjusted, and they and their parents ultimately just as often satisfied, lends some support for this policy. But in geographical terms a route is seldom recommended unless it not only reaches the destination but does so by a reasonably direct and trouble-free path. The foster parent adopters in this study did not consider their route had been trouble-free and they emphatically did not recommend it. Social workers often prefer fostering first because it postpones taking final and often painful and complicated decisions. There may be an element of self-protection alongside the stated aim of protecting the child. In effect, what may happen is the weakening of commitment and the transfer of anxiety from the social workers to the foster family and thence to the child.

Also to be weighed in the balance is the study's almost self-evident conclusion that children flourish when they are secure and feel part of a close and affectionate family. If they are 'in limbo', if they worry about the future and feel insecure in their most important relationships with adults, they do not flourish. The former foster children in this study had all become adopted children. For them the period of uncertainty was of limited duration, though sometimes it represented much of their childhood. One wonders what has happened to those foster children, placed at the same time as those studied in this sample, who were never adopted or restored to their birth parents, but instead remained in the much more nebulous relationship of foster children. Perhaps one can sum up the arguments by saying that fostering a child with a view to adoption can work out well. If it is the only available route to providing the child with really long-term family care, the risks that it entails may have to be taken and some older children may themselves prefer to be less committed at first. But there is nothing at all in this study to recommend this method over a more rapid, direct and less anxiety-provoking route when that is possible. The implication for practice is that fostering with a view to adoption, or just ordinary fostering that eventually develops into adoption, is a roundabout way of achieving the security of a permanent relationship, though it is true that with older or damaged children, such as are being placed today, the period between placement and court hearing may need to be considerably extended so that any feeling of pressure is avoided.

'Matching'

In recent years much scorn has been heaped on the concept of matching a child to his prospective adopters. The impossibility of making accurate predictions about a baby's future personality, appearance or intellectual capacity has led some people to suggest that adoptive applicants ought to be willing to accept almost any child since there is no choice in birth. The successful placement of black children in white families can also be put forward as proof that matching is at best irrelevant, and at worst positively damaging, in that it appears to collude with people's fantasies and with their unwillingness to accept the inherent differences of adoptive parenthood.

There is no question but that some of the matching exercises in the past were carried to absurd lengths, and equally true that an interracial family – certainly the antithesis of matching as far as appearance and culture are concerned – can be as close and feal as real as any other.

Nevertheless, the findings of this study are unequivocal. Both adoptive parents and their grown-up children have made it clear that a feeling of likeness is part of the feeling of kinship and that a characteristic of less than happy adoptions is a sense of difference and not belonging. The characteristics which families like to share may well be interests and values rather than physical likeness, abilities or temperament and the similarities may be the result of living together rather than anything inherent; indeed they may be matters of belief rather than actuality but none the less effective for all that. And if one thinks of adoption as a graft or transplant of a child from one family tree to another, the idea of matching in the broad sense of suitability makes sense.

The tendency to perceive likeness to oneself as 'good' and difference as 'bad' seems to be rather universal. It is interesting that we use the word 'like' to mean both 'similar' and 'pleasing'. No doubt this yearning for the comfort of similarity lies behind the pleasure expressed by both adopters and adoptees over shared characteristics. It ties in, too, with the development of identity and an acceptable self-image. Most people enjoy knowing something about their ancestors. An adopted child has to settle for himself the reality of his dual background. His task is easier if he can see some similarities in his two families to act as reference points with which to draw them together, and if he feels that his adoptive family is appropriate as well as accepting.

With the infant placements reported here, any matching had to be on the basis of background and possibly the baby's looks. In the older child adoptions being undertaken today, the 'fit' has to be on the basis of personality, life-style, mutual needs and expectations. No-one can accurately predict the chemistry of the new combination when a strange child is added to a family. Adoption workers do not have second sight. But professional responsibility must involve using every scrap of knowledge and skill available and being willing to re-examine theories and practice in the face of new evidence.

The adoptive parents' need for their child to 'get on' and be a credit to them was so marked in the study families that it clearly needs to be taken into consideration when selecting a home for a child. Traditionally, social workers have tended to look favourably on families whose expectations were moderate and realistic and there was sound sense in this. Yet the study findings about adopted people's need to achieve well for their *own* satisfaction cannot be ignored either. Most older children now being placed in substitute families are educationally retarded, and without very skilled psychological assessment it may be difficult to know how much of the retardation is due to inherently limited intellectual capacity and how much to disturbance and deprivation. If the latter, how much will be reversible? Should much more attention be paid to the remedial education needs of children joining new families and to finding activities, sports, crafts, etc., and, later, vocational training in which they can learn skills likely to increase their confidence and self-respect?

As we saw from the project families, adoptive parents often can cope remarkably well with retardation that is obvious and explicable. They may find it much more difficult to accept a general failure to achieve and can be disappointed and resentful if all their efforts to help do not restore the child to what they consider a suitable level of intellectual capacity. The short attention-span and lack of sustained interests or hobbies that are so common a mark of deprived children and adolescents may be almost inexplicable and deeply distressing to families in which a range of interests is taken for granted. This is where the matching of life-style and personality in older child placement becomes so crucial yet often so hard to manage.

Service to adoptive families
In the intervening years since the adopted people in this project were placed,

the assessment of adoptive applicants has become much more thorough. But it is only recently, since the differences between natural and adoptive parenthood have been borne in on social workers by feedback from adoptive families, that the emphasis has been placed on education for the task. This puts a further responsibility on social workers, as they need to know not only how to assess people as potential parents but also enough about the uniqueness of adoptive family life to teach it to applicants wishing to enter into this relationship with a child.

It is only as the differences in adoptive parenthood have become recognised and acknowledged that the idea of *continuing* social work service to them has become respectable. At the time the adoptions described here took place, the theory was that adoption agencies should not intrude on the families they had helped to create for fear of singling them out as unusual. As we have seen, a small percentage of project parents saw the possibility of the agency being helpful when adolescent problems arose and a few who had not been able to discuss background with their children saw the possibility of the agency being helpful by handling this for them. While it obviously would not be appropriate for the agency to take over this parental function, the findings about the problems many of these families had in discussing adoption are disturbing. They are another link in a growing chain of evidence which is now strong enough to require a genuine and profound re-think of adoption agencies' post-placement responsibilities. It is clearly important that voluntary and statutory agencies alike should take seriously the wording of the Children Act, 1975, which sees help to adoptive families as an integral part of any agency's adoption services.

Before a child joins a family, discussions about the need to accept and discuss a child's background in the years ahead are bound to seem remote and theoretical, and during the early months after placement the new parents are so busy taking on their role and making the child their own that it is psychologically almost impossible for them to grapple with problems of future telling. By the time they are ready to deal with this and in a mood to value and use help, the agency has long since closed the case. In the past decade we have seen a few agencies institute discussion groups for adoptive parents and these usually have proved valuable. They are quite time-consuming because there may be a snowball effect. When groups of parents come together at the time the children are entering school, they tend to ask to meet again later to share experiences and learn from each other, and this is as it should be, for it is the adolescent years that they are likely to find most difficult to cope with. Though the value of post-placement services is seldom challenged today, there are still only a few agencies which provide them in a systematic way and fewer still which offer this service for other than their own adopters. Judging from the anxieties displayed by the families in the study, there must be thousands of parents deeply worried about the new freedom of adult adopted people to gain access to their original birth records. There may be many adoptees, too, who would like this access but do not feel able to ask their adoptive parents for the basic information necessary to apply for the certificate.

It will be a difficult task not only to establish the necessary services but to persuade adoptive families to use them. As their comments to the project interviewers showed, many of the parents in this study made it clear that they would be ashamed to ask for help because it would look like failure. Too many families as well as too many social workers have equated problems with failure, apparently forgetting that for any family to be problem-free for any length of time is quite unusual. A new approach will be needed and some very good public relations work, too, if adoptive parents are going to accept as a matter of course that they probably will need to come back from time to time over the years to consult agency staff and, above all, other adoptive parents about the special tasks they all face.

TO SUM UP

Although the study's findings are not dramatic they certainly are encouraging. When they are surprising it is usually a matter of degree or because an old idea is shown up in a new light. Nor do the experiences of the project families provide a clear pattern or a formula for success. Rather, they demonstrate again the extraordinary individuality of the human situation, the varying responses people make to rather similar circumstances. They are further proof of the importance of agencies avoiding rigid rules and policies while not throwing overboard all the practice wisdom accumulated over the years. Attitudes and feelings are always more important than facts when families are being artificially created through the process of adoption. No doubt this is why a few of those we studied had failed quite badly even though on the face of it everything appeared to be in their favour, and others had triumphed over immense personal and practical problems.

Appendix A

———◆———

SOME DO'S AND DON'TS FROM ADOPTIVE PARENTS

Parents in the study were asked whether from their own experience they would recommend adopting a child and what advice they would give to anyone considering adoption. Although 15 per cent of the 160 families felt their own experience had been unsatisfactory and disappointing, only 3 per cent felt they could not recommend adoption to others. The remainder of those who were disappointed believed they had just been unlucky. All other families in the project recommended it, though 29 of them did so with some reservation or condition attached.

Almost everyone had some advice to give to anyone considering adoption. Many felt they could recommend it on the basis of their own 'lucky' experience, but that in giving advice they should warn prospective adopters about pitfalls they had heard of from others. Following is some of the advice they would like to give to adoptive applicants. It reflects a wide spectrum of opinion. Much of it is good advice, some of it is bad and more of it is conflicting.

Make sure any children already in the family will accept the adopted child.

Think ahead to beyond the baby years to when the problems start.

Take only one child or, if two, then from similar backgrounds.

Take two or more so you won't spoil the child or have all your eggs in one basket if one doesn't turn out well.

Foster a child for a few months to see if you get attached.

Don't consider fostering at any price.

Be sure you want the child, so he won't feel put aside and rejected when you tire of him.

Be prepared to do your utmost; adoption isn't easy.

You should both really like and understand children and both really want to adopt.

Adoptive parents need to be able to communicate their feelings to each other about things as they arise.

Don't adopt just because you want to rescue or help a child; be sure you want the child for his own sake.

Don't do it just to boost your own ego.

Attempt it only if you have knowledge of child development.

It is a big commitment, so be prepared for responsibility.

Be sure to watch for background, as what is in the father is in the son.

Once you have got them they are what you make of them.

It is best to have no rigid feelings of what it will be like, but be interested in whatever develops.

How the child turns out may not be your responsibility, but due to genetic endowment.

Heredity is important, but the way you bring them up is what counts most.

It is best not to know anything about the background.

Be sure to understand that upbringing plays only a small part in the outcome.

No matter what happens you will reap rewards, because every child brings so much love. (This was from parents whose adopted child had to be hospitalised because of severe mental retardation.)

The children don't always develop as you expect.

Adopt only if you are sure and willing to take a risk. It is worth the gamble.

Make the child your own and never think of him as another's child.

Tell him early and be open about adoption.

Tell the child early, then forget he is adopted.

Tell him he is adopted but nothing about his background, and don't refer to it again once he understands.

Consider the child your own and commit yourself to him fully.

If you treat them as your own and forget about adoption you will feel for them just as for a natural child.

Don't expect a child to turn out to be absolutely marvellous and do everything just as you did.

Don't expect to live your life through the child.

Forget he is adopted and don't blame everything on adoption.

Appendix B

◆

GUIDE TO INTERVIEW WITH ADOPTIVE PARENTS

DEMOGRAPHIC INFORMATION

Is family still intact?
Age of child at time of any break in family.
Adoptive mother's employment outside the home before child aged 12.
Physical and mental health of family since the adoption.
Status, sex and age difference of children who joined family later.

OUTCOME OF THE ADOPTION FROM PARENTS' POINT OF VIEW

Anything they particularly want to tell us.
Parents' overall assessment of experience with this child.
Nature of their early experience with this child:

(a) basis on which child was received into family (adoption or fostering);
(b) view of advantage or disadvantage of this method of placement;
(c) any contact between adopters and natural mother? Their view of this;
(d) how well did this child fit their idea of child they wanted;
(e) any early doubts?
(f) nature of child and adopters' early adjustment to each other.

In what ways has the experience been satisfying to them? In what ways disappointing?
To what do they attribute any problems with the child?
Would it have been helpful to have met with other adopters to discuss problems of mutual concern?
Would they have liked more help from the placement agency?
Would they recommend adoption to others?
What advice would they give to someone adopting a child?
Their views on heredity and environment in relation to adoption outcome.

RELATIONSHIP WITH THE CHILD

Their general tone in speaking of this child.
Who made decisions about the child's upbringing?
Who was emotionally closest to child while growing up?
Closeness in relationship with child over the years.
View of this child's place in the family group.

Attitude of siblings over the years.
Attitude of grandparents and community over the years.
Do parents feel they really understood this child?
Their relationship with child while growing up.
Areas of anxiety or tension in relationship with child while growing up.
Degree of each parent's involvement with the child and how this compared with their
involvement with other children in the family.
Degree of parental control they exerted.
Overall atmosphere in home while child growing up there.

COMMUNICATION WITH CHILD CONCERNING ADOPTION

Timing and circumstances of disclosure of fostering or adoptive relationship, what
was told, what was withheld.
Child's reaction then and later to the revelation.
Has child ever asked for or seemed to want more information?
Did parents wish they had been given more information or did they know some-
thing they wished they had not been told?
How often was adoption or background mentioned over years and who most often
initiated it?
Parents' ease and comfort over the years in discussing this.
Did anything in child's background make discussion harder?
Has child made any effort to contact or learn more about natural parents?

THE CHILD, AS DESCRIBED BY THE ADOPTIVE PARENTS

Word they think best describes this child.
Traits they have liked most in the child.
Traits they have liked least in the child?
Do they think the child was like them in some way? How?
Ways in which they had a difficult time with the child:

(a) medical problems and how they were handled;
(b) developmental problems and how they were handled;
(c) behaviour, personality, emotional problems and how they were handled,
including any conflict with the law.

Relationship with peers while growing up.
Age child left school and highest educational attainment.
How well child fulfilled parents' educational aspirations.

THE PRESENT

Child's present marital status.
Child's present living arrangements.
Child's present means of financial support.
Child's present occupation and length of present employment.
Parents' view of child's work adjustment.

Parents' view of child's sexual adjustment, e.g. happily married, promiscuous, etc.

Parents' view of child's use of opportunities offered.

Parents' view of child's present self-concept.

Parents' view of how child values other people.

How parents think child views his experience of adoption.

Parents' view of their own relationship with child.

Parents' predominant current feeling towards this child, e.g. pride, disappointment, hurt, rejection, etc.

Do they see this child as their 'own' son or daughter?

Child's likely response to being asked to take part in the study.

Parents' view of whether the child should be invited to take part.

Appendix C

---◆---

GUIDE TO INTERVIEW WITH ADULT ADOPTEES

DEMOGRAPHIC INFORMATION

Present marital status.
Present living arrangements.
Present employment.
Length of present employment.

RELATIONSHIP WITH ADOPTIVE FAMILY OVER THE YEARS

Overall view of the experience of growing up adopted.
View of how much he is like adoptive family.
Feeling of closeness to adoptive family while growing up.
Relationship with other children in adoptive family.
View of his place within the family group.
View of kind of care received.
View of intensity and consistency of parental control.
View of adoptive parents' expectations of him.
View of freedom of choice while growing up.
View of emotional tone of the home while growing up there.

DISCLOSURE OF ADOPTIVE STATUS AND RELATED INFORMATION

Age and circumstances when learned adopted.
Reaction to learning of adoption.
Any period of doubt or uncertainty?
Degree of satisfaction with information received.
What information was received?
Frequency of discussion with adoptive parents about this over the years.
Freedom and comfort in discussing subject with adoptive parents?
Attitude to adoptive parents knowing or not knowing natural mother.
View of adoptive parents' attitude to background.
Which does adoptee now feel are his 'real' parents?

CURRENT PERSONAL AND SOCIAL ADJUSTMENT

Own view of use he has made of opportunities.
Own satisfaction with his present life.
View of life and the world.
Current relationship with each adoptive parent.
Attitude to natural parents.
Current relationship with friends, colleagues or workmates.
Attitude to marriage and children.
How describes self.
Anything else adoptee wants to tell us re. his experience as an adopted person.
View of being asked to take part in this study.

REFERENCES

Addis, Robina, Salzberger, F., and Rabl, E. (1955), *A Survey Based on Adoption Case Records* (London: National Association for Mental Health).

Bamford, Terry (1977), 'Why the poor pay more', *Social Work Today*, vol. 9, no. 5, p. 5.

Bohman, Michael (1970), *Adopted Children and their Families* (Stockholm: Proprius).

Borgotta, E. F., and Fanshel, David (1965), *Behaviour Characteristics of Children Known to Psychiatric Outpatient Clinics* (New York: Child Welfare League of America).

Brenner, Ruth (1951), *A Follow Up Study of Adoptive Families* (New York: Child Adoption Research Committee).

Central Statistical Office, Office of Population Censuses and Surveys, *Annual Abstract of Statistics 1976* (London: HMSO).

Fanshel, David (1972), *Far from the Reservation* (Metuchen, NJ: Scarecrow Press).

Fogelman, K. (1976), *Britain's 16 Year Olds* (London: National Children's Bureau).

Gibson, Colin (1974), 'The association between divorce and social class in England and Wales', *British Journal of Sociology*, vol. 25, no. 1, pp. 79–93.

Grow, L. J., and Shapiro, D. (1974), *Black Children - White Parents* (New York: Child Welfare League of America).

Hoopes, J. L., Sherman, E. A., Lawder, E. A., Andrews, R. G., and Lower, K. D. (1969), *A Follow-Up Study of Adoptions, (Vol. II): Post Placement Functioning of Adopted Children* (New York: Child Welfare League of America).

Humphrey, M., and Ounsted, C. (1963), 'Adoptive families referred for psychiatric advice, Part I: the children', *British Journal of Psychiatry*, vol. 109, pp. 599–608.

Jackson, Barbara (1975), *Family Experiences in Interracial Adoption* (London: Association of British Adoption and Fostering Agencies).

Jaffee, Benson (1974), 'Adoptive outcome: A two generation view', *Child Welfare* (USA), vol. 53, no. 4, pp. 211–24.

Jaffee, B., and Fanshel, D. (1970), *How They Fared in Adoption: A Follow-up Study* (New York: Columbia University Press).

Kadushin, Alfred (1970), *Adopting Older Children* (New York and London: Columbia University Press).

Kadushin, Alfred, and Seidl, Fred (1971), 'Adoption failure', *Social Work* (USA), vol. 16, no. 3, pp. 32–8.

Kornitzer, Margaret (1968), *Adoption and Family Life* (London: Putnam).

Krugman, Dorothy (1964), 'Reality in adoption', *Child Welfare*, vol. 43, pp. 349–58.

Lawder, E. A., Lower, K. D., Andrews, R. G., Sherman, E. A., and Hill, J. G. (1969), *A Follow-Up Study of Adoptions: Post Placement Functioning of Adoption Families* (New York: Child Welfare League of America).

Leeding, Alfred (1977) 'Access to birth records', *Adoption and Fostering*, no. 89, pp. 19–25.

McWhinnie, A. M. (1967), *Adopted Children - How They Grow Up: A Study of their Adjustment as Adults* (London: Routledge & Kegan Paul).

National Federation of Adoptive Parent Associations (1976), 'What is the attitude of adopted youths towards adoption?', *International Child Welfare Review*, nos. 30/1, pp. 146–7.

Nicholls, R. H., and Wray, F. A. (1935), *The History of the Foundling Hospital* (London: Oxford University Press).

Peller, L. E. (1961), 'About telling the child about his adoption', *Bulletin of the Philadelphia Association for Psychoanalysis*, 11, pp. 145–54.

Peller, L. E. (1962), 'Further comments on adoption', *Bulletin of the Philadelphia Association for Psychoanalysis*, 13, pp. 1–14.

Pringle, M. L. K., Butler, N. R., and Davie, R. (1966), *11,000 Seven-year-olds* (London: Longman).

Raynor, Lois (1970), *Adoption of Non-White Children* (London: Allen & Unwin).

Rosner, Gertrude (1961), *Crisis of Self-Doubt* (New York: Child Welfare League of America).

Rowe, Jane (1970), 'The realities of adoptive parenthood', *Child Adoption*, no. 59, pp. 23–29.

Rutter, Michael (1970), 'Psychological development – predictions from infancy', *Journal of Child Psychology and Psychiatry*, vol. 11, pp. 49–62.

Rutter, Michael, Tizard, Jack, and Whitmore, Kingsley (1970), *Education, Health and Behaviour* (London: Longman).

Sants, H. J. (1964), 'Genealogical bewilderment in children with substitute parents', *British Journal of Medical Psychology*, Vol. 37, pp. 133–41.

Schecter, M. D. (1960), 'Observations on adopted children', *American Medical Association Archives of General Psychiatry*, 3, pp. 45–56.

Schecter, M. D., Carlson, P. V., Simmons, J. Q., and Work, H. H. (1964), 'Emotional problems in the adoptee', *Archives of General Psychiatry*, 10, pp. 37–46.

Seglow, J., Pringle, M. L. K., and Wedge, P. (1972), *Growing Up Adopted* (London: National Foundation for Educational Research).

Shaw, Lulie (1953), 'Following up adoptions', *British Journal of Psychiatric Social Work*, vol. 8, pp. 14–21.

Simon, R. J., and Altstein, M. (1977), *Transracial Adoption* (New York: Wiley).

Skeels, H. M., and Harms, I. (1948), 'Children with inferior social histories, their mental development in adoptive homes', *Journal of Genetic Psychology*, 72, pp. 283–94.

Skodak, M., and Skeels, H. M. (1949), 'A final follow up study of 100 adopted children', *Journal of Genetic Psychology*, 75, pp. 85–125.

Stone, F. H. (1969), 'Adoption and identity', *Child Adoption*, no. 58, pp. 17–28.

Sweeney, D. M., Gasbarro, D. T., and Gluck, M. R. (1963), 'A descriptive study of adopted children seen in a child guidance center', *Child Welfare* (USA), vol. 42, pp. 345–9.

Theis, Sophie Van S. (1924), *How Foster Children Turn Out* (New York: State Charities Aid Association).

Thompson, E. J., and Peretz, Jane (eds) (1977) *Social Trends*, no. 8 (London: HMSO).

Tizard, Barbara (1977), *Adoption: A Second Chance* (London: Open Books).

Triseliotis, John (1973), *In Search of Origins* (London and Boston: Routledge & Kegan Paul).

Triseliotis, John (1974), 'Identity and adoption', *Child Adoption*, no. 78 pp. 27–34.

Witmer, H. L., Herzog, E., Weinstein, E. A., and Sullivan, M. E. (1963), *Independent Adoptions* (New York, Russell Sage Foundation).

Wittenborn, J. R. (1957), *The Placement of Adoptive Children* (Springfield, Ill.: Thomas).

INDEX

Milton Keynes UK
Ingram Content Group UK Ltd.
UKHW022050141024
449569UK00031B/1569